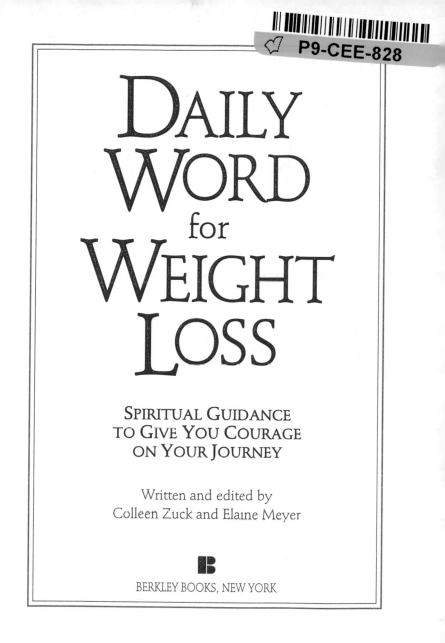

DAILY WORD for WEIGHT LOSS

SPIRITUAL GUIDANCE TO GIVE YOU COURAGE ON YOUR JOURNEY

Written and edited by
Colleen Zuck and Elaine Meyer

BERKLEY BOOKS, NEW YORK

PUBLISHER'S NOTE

Every effort has been made to ensure that the information contained in this book is complete and accurate. However, neither the pubisher nor the author is engaged in rendering professional advice or services to the individual reader. The ideas, procedures, and suggestions contained in this book are not intended as a substitute for consulting with your physician. All matters regarding your health require medical supervision. Neither the author nor the publisher shall be liable or responsible for any loss or damage allegedly arising from any information or suggestions in this book.

A Berkley Book
Published by The Berkley Publishing Group
A division of Penguin Putnam Inc.
375 Hudson Street
New York, New York 10014

Cover design by Joanna Williams.
Cover illustration by Dave Cutler.

PRINTING HISTORY
Rodale Press hardcover edition / February 2002
Berkley trade paperback edition / January 2003

Visit our website at
www.penguinputnam.com

Library of Congress Cataloging-in-Publication Data

Zuck, Colleen.
Daily word for weight loss : spiritual guidance to give you courage on your journey / written and edited by Collen Zuck and Elaine Meyer.
p. cm.
Originally published: Emmaus, Pa. : Rodale, 2002.
ISBN 0-425-18827-2
1. Weight loss—Religious aspects—Christianity. I. Meyer, Elaine.
II. Title.
RM222.2 .Z796 2003
646.7'5—dc21 2002028219

PRINTED IN THE UNITED STATES OF AMERICA

10 9 8 7 6 5 4 3 2 1

An Invitation

Daily Word is the magazine of Silent Unity, a worldwide prayer ministry now in its second century of service. Silent Unity believes that:

- *all people are sacred*
- *God is present in all situations*
- *everyone is worthy of love, peace, health, and prosperity*

Supported by free-will offerings, Silent Unity prays with all who ask for prayer. Every prayer request is held in absolute confidence. You are invited to contact Silent Unity 24 hours a day, any day of the year.

Write: Silent Unity, 1901 NW Blue Parkway
Unity Village, MO 64065-0001
Or call: (816) 969-2000 Fax: (816) 251-3554
www.unityworldhq.org

There's More!

If you enjoy these inspirational messages, you may wish to subscribe to *Daily Word* magazine and receive a fresh, contemporary, uplifting message for each day of the month. With its inclusive, universal language, this pocket-size magazine is a friend to millions of people around the world.

For a free sample copy or for subscription information regarding *Daily Word* in English (regular and large-type editions) or in Spanish, please write:

Silent Unity, 1901 NW Blue Parkway
Unity Village, MO 64065-0001
Or call: (800) 669-0282 Fax: (816) 251-3554
www.unityworldhq.org

List of Articles

Acknowledgments

This book was made possible through the team effort of the *Daily Word* editors and the dedicated and talented Silent Unity Composition Department: Peggy Pifer, Debbie Cameron, Sharon King, and Candi Foster.

Introduction

You may be questioning, "What makes this book different from hundreds of other books on weight loss?" First of all, it is not a diet plan; it is a whole-self plan for a journey of healthful living. Between the covers of this book, you will discover that by uniting the power of your whole self—spirit, mind, and body—you can lose weight, and even more important, you can maintain that weight loss over a lifetime.

Following the whole-self plan requires a commitment by you, but it is one that will enrich the way you look and feel and act. With your whole self involved, you are in control of your life, of what you eat, and of how often you exercise.

By now you probably know that willpower alone will not bring about the results you desire. Neither will the best diet plan ever conceived. Yet when you apply the God-power within you that is waiting to empower you, you will strengthen your willpower and you intuitively will know what to do to lose weight and to achieve greater health of mind and body.

What can you expect to learn and experience from reading this book? Expect to be successful, because your expectations are powerful thoughts that help you create your experiences. There is life and intelligence within the very cells of your body that listen to and respond to what you think and say.

Expect to be inspired. The word *inspire* has its roots in the idea of Spirit literally breathing life into a creation. You were created for life, but you may need to be refreshed by a greater awareness of God, a breath of divine inspiration, so that you will move forward in becoming healthier and happier. Throughout the following pages, you will be reminded that you can, for you are never alone in any moment of the day and night. Because the spirit of God lives within you, you are offered constant encouragement to be the healthy, happy person that God created you to be.

How many of us have been caught in the cycle of losing and then regaining 20 to 25 pounds over the years? It's time to break that cycle. We believe that in *Daily Word for Weight Loss*, you will find inspiration, motivation, and practical tips and information that will help you break free from old, negative thoughts and habits and establish new, positive thoughts and habits.

How to Use This Book

You are beginning a journey on which you will be making daily discoveries of what does and does not fit into your goal of losing weight and maintaining your weight loss. How often you read from this book—whether it's every day or once a week—will depend on you and your needs. However, the more inspired, informed, and motivated you are, the more easily you will cope with large and small challenges along your path. You may choose to start at the beginning and read some every day. The theme for the first half of the book is weight loss; for the second half, maintaining that weight loss. We believe the book will be a continuing resource for you whenever you need inspiration.

1. Stories: True-life stories of seven women are featured. The women share how they have dealt with success, setbacks, and recovery. Some are still on the journey to their weight-loss goals. Others have reached their goals and are maintaining them. They offer different approaches to taking off weight and some practical information about what worked for them. Tamara Guilliams's story reveals how she accomplished her goal of losing weight—a total weight loss that is equivalent to what a professional football linebacker might weigh! Susan Smith Jones provides information based on her years as a fitness instructor and health advocate. She provides the answers to such questions as, "Why does drinking more water help relieve that feeling of bloat?"

2. Daily messages: These are prayerful, practical, and powerful messages of support for you—no matter where you are on your journey. They are written in the singular voice of you, the individual reader. They are true for you, because they are true for each child of God. Reading the affirmation, practical application of a divine principle, and a Bible verse, you are opening your mind and life to great possibilities.

3. Meditations: Each guided meditation will jump start you in getting in touch with inner spiritual power and in using it to enhance the way you look and feel. Through these pages you truly do unite mind, body, and soul with Spirit so that you experience a wholeness that is so palpable, so powerful that you will succeed in whatever you desire to accomplish.

4. Journal pages: On these pages, you will be your own fitness coach. No one knows you better than you know yourself. A thought-provoking statement will encourage you to capture what helped you most in achieving weight loss, greater peace of mind, or anything else that has enriched you on your journey.

5. Tips: You will be offered information and tools that help bring about good results. Sometimes it's one event that can be a detour from weeks of good behavior. These tips will help you get back on track.

Know that the prayers of Silent Unity are with you on your journey. We behold you filled with light and making steady progress each day of your journey to greater health and wholeness.

—The Editors

Research at Vanderbilt University shows that overweight people who usually skipped breakfast lost an average of 17 pounds over 3 months after they started eating breakfast. In addition, they were better able to keep the weight off. Why? Breakfast eaters snack less frequently and are less hungry during the remainder of the day.

♠

SOURCE: *American Institute for Preventive Medicine (2001)*

Looking at the Real Me

By Tamara Guilliams

The 367 pounds I have lost is not a result of a special diet plan; I believe it is the ongoing result of a healing that began within the depths of my soul 5 years ago.

Before that healing took place, I had been extremely self-critical, believing that anything negative in my life was somehow my fault. The driving force behind that self-criticism was something that had happened to me at age 11, something horrible that I kept secret from my family and everyone else: I had been raped by three neighborhood boys. From that point on, I began to sabotage my own life by being self-destructive. By the time I was a teenager, I was into alcohol and drugs, trying to numb the pain I felt over being abused and becoming increasingly overweight.

Although I always had been chubby, after I married and had two children, my weight ballooned to 550 pounds. I slept sitting in a recliner because I could no longer breathe lying down. I had to depend on my children to put my shoes on because I could not reach my feet. My husband and I had been married for almost 15 years, but it was an unhealthy situation for both of us, because we fed off each other's self-destructiveness.

Then in a very short period of time, my father died, my husband asked for a divorce, and I had pneumonia and liver problems. Because of the excess weight, my body seemed to be shutting down. All this was bad enough, but my whole world came crashing down around me when my doctor told me that if my health continued to decline, I had only about 6 months to live.

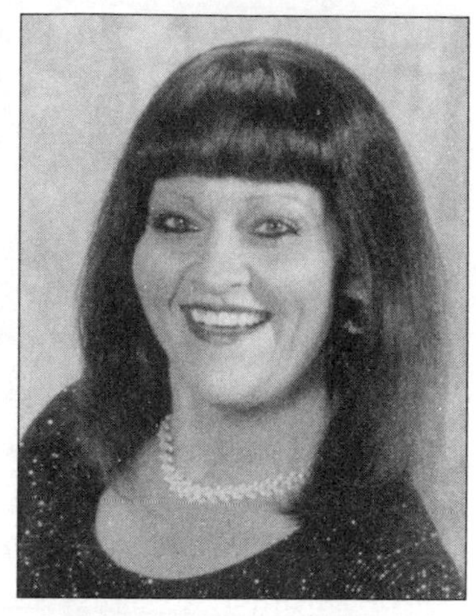

I spent the next several days at home with the shades drawn, sobbing and feeling sorry for myself. At one point, I needed a fresh supply of tissues to wipe away a flood of new tears. Walking to the bathroom for the tissues, I passed a mirror. I caught a glimpse of someone, but I was certain it was not me that I saw. Turning back to the mirror, I heard an inner voice saying, "Look at the real you."

As I stared into the mirror, I felt as if I were looking past my image into my very soul to see that child of God I truly was. Suddenly I felt a renewal of strength come over me, a surge of spiritual awareness. As a child of God, I prayed to be healed of the unhappiness I had held inside me for so long. Those first few prayers were pleas: "God, let me live one more day! I promise I will do something in this world that will make a difference!" and "Let me see one more sunrise!"

Then when I woke up in the morning to see another sunrise, I was filled with gratitude, saying, "Thank You, God." I started to look at people and nature with a new appreciation for all life. I loved and appreciated my children more than ever. Before I had been depressed; now I felt excited about life.

From the moment that I had the experience in the mirror, I stopped drinking and doing drugs. And I started losing weight. Working within at my soul level, I was healing my body. I continued to do mirror work. Daily I spoke into the mirror, to that child of God that I now knew I was. I saw my true self and also recognized that the presence of God was within me.

When someone had been unkind or uncaring toward me during the day, I looked into the mirror that evening and reassured myself: "As a child of God, I deserve to be loved and I desire to express love toward others." This kind of affirmation strengthened me spiritually, emotionally, and even physically.

I was no longer suppressing my feelings by allowing food to keep me numb about life. I continued with my mirror work, looking at myself and saying, "I love you just the way you are." I prepared and ate food for someone I loved and cared about. I wanted to be as loving and kind and supportive toward myself, toward others, and toward the world as I could be.

Family and friends started telling me: "Your clothes seem to fit you a lot looser," and "You are so radiant; there is a different energy coming from you." I recognized changes in myself and felt joyous about them.

My mother, who was working at Unity School of Christianity, suggested that I take a couple of classes taught there. She believed that these spiritually enriching classes would help in my healing. So I signed up for the "Life of Prayer" and "Lessons in Truth" classes. I felt awkward walking into the classroom that first day, wondering, "Will I fit into a chair? Will the other students stare at me?"

Once in the classroom, I did have to pull two chairs together in order to sit down, but much to my surprise, no one was staring at me. People were smiling and talking and greeting each other with hugs. They seemed so accepting and loving. For the first time in a long time, I felt as if I fit in with a group of people. We learned together, and we prayed for one another.

One of my assignments was to lead the class in a 5-minute meditation. Immediately afterward I didn't remember what I had said in those 5 minutes, but I did realize that I was in touch with the spirit of God within me. Meditation became a part of my day, every day—for

30 minutes in the morning and 30 minutes to an hour in the evening. Sometimes I would go outside and simply breathe in the air and listen to the wind blowing and birds singing. I realized that as I became still, I was peaceful, and I could visualize what I would look like if I were completely healthy and whole. I began to make that visualization a reality by what I did and what I ate.

Following in my mother's footsteps, I applied and was accepted for a job at Unity. Being in a workplace that was saturated with prayer, I realized greater healing and greater weight loss.

I realized that something bad had happened to me as a girl of 11, but I had not caused it to happen. Even though those teenage boys had hurt me, it was up to me to stop punishing myself and ruining my health by overeating. My extra weight had served as a barrier that kept me separated from others. Because I feared being hurt in some way, I had literally manifested walls with my body that said, "Stay away!"

Finally able to talk to family and friends about what had happened, I was reassured and comforted by their love and compassion toward me. Each time I would go back for a check-up, I amazed the doctors with how much weight I had lost. My sons called me the incredible shrinking woman, and I cherished each encouraging remark anyone made.

I am a new person now—in the way I look and feel.

But most important I realize that I am a child of God who deserves the blessings of God. Regaining my health and self-esteem has not been easy. I had surgery to remove a malignant tumor and then went through 20 radiation treatments. At first, I questioned, "Why me?" but the answer came, "You have the power and strength to face this challenge." And I did.

I have held onto what I had discovered in a mirror 5 years ago: I am a creation of God, and God doesn't make mistakes. Everything that has happened in my life has helped shape me into who I am today, and I don't have regrets, because I love who I am.

Each one of us needs to look at our lives but not waste time regretting anything. Forgiving everyone and everything, we are able to love who we are. Because we truly do love ourselves, we bring out strengths, qualities, and talents that we never realized we had.

Challenges happen in life, and we can look at them as either stumbling blocks or as stepping stones. Choosing to recognize ourselves as children of God and to love who we are, just as we are, we understand that challenges are stepping stones that move us forward in life and forward on our spiritual journey of discovery.

Today's Message
Guidance

——◆——

God guides me in knowing what is absolutely best for me in losing weight.

There is an abundance of advice, suggestions, and information available to me about how to lose weight; however, is some of it, any of it, right for me?

The question I ask myself is this: "What would God have me do to succeed?" Seeking the guidance of my Creator, I will know what is absolutely best for me, because it will fit my unique needs.

God is my guide to all that blesses me and to all the ways I can be a blessing to myself and others. I receive divine guidance in the quiet of meditation and in the whir of activity. Divine guidance is a certain knowing of what to do and how to go about doing it.

God honors me by giving me all that I need to know to be successful. I honor God by giving my best in following divine guidance. Ours is a partnership of Creator and created, a relationship established between God and me.

"But surely, God is my helper;
the Lord is the upholder of my life."
—Psalms 54:4

Today's Message
Healthy Start

***As each new day dawns,
I make a healthy new start.***

The dawning of each new day is an opportunity for me to make a healthy start. As I begin anew, I turn to God, who is my unfailing source of help. God is my faithful companion and friend, my help in living a happy, healthy life.

A healthy start begins in communication with God. I quiet my thoughts, and as I do, God tenderly nurtures and encourages me.

By beginning my day with God, I give my attention to God and the sacredness of my own body. I then treat my body with the respect and care it deserves, taking an important step to greater health.

My daily communion with God fills me with new resolve and helps me develop an unflagging commitment to eat sensibly and exercise wisely. Reinforcing good habits, I make a healthy start that places me firmly on a pathway to success.

**"By the tender mercy of our God,
the dawn from on high will break upon us."
—Luke 1:78**

TODAY'S MESSAGE

Being Myself

—◆—

I express my true self by being loving and wise and by using good judgment.

I have often heard the expression, "Just be yourself." Yet what does this really mean?

When I practice being myself, I am being true to who and what I am—a child of God. Because I am a spiritual being, made in the image of God, I know that my true self is strong, whole, and free.

I am true to myself when I express the qualities of God within me, such as love, wisdom, and good judgment, in all that I say and do.

I express the love of God within me to others and also remember to love myself. I let the wisdom of God guide me in making choices that are right for me, and I use good judgment in how I evaluate and value myself.

I practice seeing myself as God sees me—whole and perfect in every way. I can do anything my true self desires to do when I rely on God to guide me and help me.

"Clothe yourselves with the new self, created according to the likeness of God in true righteousness and holiness."
—Ephesians 4:24

Today's Message

Comfort

God sustains me and comforts me, satisfying the hunger of my soul.

I can be of great help to myself by knowing what truly comforts me. This is important, because in the past I may have felt that I could rely on food as my comfort, but the more I tried to find comfort in food, the more uncomfortable I felt.

Every day I am learning more and more about what is for my well-being and what is not. One thing I do know is that God is my comfort, no matter what I am going through. Even a brief prayer eases tension in my body and allows me to relax. As I say God's name silently when facing a decision-making situation, I recognize that the Creator of all life is with me to sustain me and comfort me.

My comfort is not in what I eat or how much I eat. My relationship with God is my comfort, a comfort that sustains me in every situation. Yes, God truly does satisfy the hunger of my soul.

"And he will guide them to springs of the water of life, and God will wipe away every tear from their eyes."
—Revelation 7:17

Today's Message

Goals

—◆—

Maintaining a positive self-image helps me move forward in accomplishing my goal.

Feeling good mentally, emotionally, and physically requires an investment by me. So I set goals that keep me moving in a positive direction.

As I move forward in meeting my goals, I remember to do something for myself that acknowledges my good efforts—something that gives me pleasure and relaxes me. I may make time in my schedule to take a walk, read a book, or relax in a bubble bath—something that rewards me for even what seems like a small achievement that kept me on track.

If at any point along the way I seem to be falling short of my goal, I do not berate or punish myself. I am a child of God, happy, healthy, and filled with self-assurance.

I hold to my goal and maintain a positive self-image, all the while remembering what my expectations are and giving thanks that God can lead me to even greater ones.

"You guide me with your counsel."
—Psalms 73:24

TODAY'S MESSAGE

Eating Right

Eating in healthy, nourishing ways energizes me with youthful exuberance.

There are many healthy, nutritious, and filling vegetables and fruits available to me, so I fortify my body by including selections from both these food groups in my diet.

Although I may find it easy to eat the right food in the right amounts when I am at home or at the office, I may not find it so easy when I am observing special occasions with friends and loved ones. At such times, I may feel an obligation to eat foods that I would not normally eat.

If the temptation to overeat begins to lurk in my thoughts, I picture how I look fit and trim. Visualizing what I am working to achieve helps me to handle those difficult situations. Eating healthy foods leaves me feeling energized and youthful. Adding exercise to my schedule brings me positive results that show when I step on the scales.

**"I will strengthen you,
I will help you."
—Isaiah 41:10**

MEDITATION

Blessing My Body

Relaxing in the presence of God,
I bless my body.

In a few moments of meditation, I relax and receive a greater realization of God's presence within me and the sacredness of my body.

Gently and slowly, I move my thoughts from whatever is happening around me to the presence of God at the core of my being. Quiet and still, I get in touch with the sacredness within me. I feel a vital, palpable connection with my Creator.

I move beyond simply being at ease to a realization of complete serenity. I am a holy being, because the spirit of God is within me. God's spirit lives out through me as health and well-being. The realization of God's presence spreads throughout my body, blessing my digestive system, organs, and nerves. My body serves me well, and I am open to ways that I can bless my body by nourishing it with food, rest, activity, and prayer.

"Do you not know that your body is a temple of the Holy Spirit within you, which you have from God, and that you are not your own?"
—1 Corinthians 6:19

◆ *Journal* ◆

Date: ______________________________

My weight: ______________________________

Achieving weight-loss goals
in steps inspires me to meet
my long-term goals.

My short-term goals are ______________________________

____

____

____

____

____

____

____

____

____

____

Today's Message

Breath of Life

—◆—

As I breathe deeply and evenly, the life of God within me responds as refreshing energy.

Because I recognize God daily in my life, I live my life as a prayer, praying with my thoughts, words, and actions. I try never to take anything for granted, including the very air that I breathe, for I am constantly refreshed by the life-sustaining activity of breathing in and out.

With each breath, I breathe in the life of God. As I breathe deeply and evenly, I close my eyes and ears to outer activities and feel the life of God within me responding as energy. Feelings of doubt or inadequacy are swept from my mind and quickly replaced with thoughts of peace.

I breathe in deeply again and bless my body with life-giving energy. I am invigorated and revitalized! I thank God for the breath of life, for the healthy food that nourishes me, and for another day in which to live my life fully and completely.

"The God who made the world and everything in it . . . gives to all mortals life and breath and all things."
—Acts 17:24–25

TODAY'S MESSAGE

Turning Point

At every turning point, God is with me as my sure and steady guide.

Life is not usually a straight-ahead journey on level ground. There are hills and valleys, twists and turns. And there are crossroads also.

Perhaps every day is a crossroads at which I ask myself, "Do I continue on my way toward the same goal, or do I turn toward another goal?" I may not come up with an answer immediately, but when I ask God and truly listen for an answer, I will receive it. It may not come in that moment, but it will come.

The answer will be one that keeps me moving toward the light of a brighter day and, concerning my weight, to a lighter day. At every turning point, I move on to make further progress.

I may come to many crossroads, but God is with me to point the way and to say, "Take My hand, beloved; this is the way."

"And your life will be brighter than the noonday; its darkness will be like the morning. And you will have confidence, because there is hope."
—Job 11:17–18

Today's Message
In the Silence

In the silence, God waits for me.

In the silence of my soul, there is a sacred place where I go to heal myself of the hurtful words or actions of others. God alone waits for me and welcomes me home.

The silence is a retreat where I go to rest in the presence of God. There I am relieved of all concern, for I am sheltered by divine love and acceptance.

In the stillness of my soul, God encourages me to become as a child—free of doubt—so that I view the world with childlike wonder.

Ready to begin anew, I leave the silence refreshed and revitalized. I once again view the world through the eyes of a child and accept the good that awaits me. The harsh words and actions of others have no power over me, because I am enfolded in the love and care of God. I am at peace.

**"Blessed be the Lord,
for he has wondrously shown
his steadfast love to me."
—Psalms 31:21**

Today's Message

Resilient Spirit

I am resilient, because God's spirit within me gives me great flexibility.

How gracefully a willow sways in summer's gentle breezes. Yet when the ice or snow of winter weighs down its branches, it appears that they will break and the tree will be permanently damaged. But appearances are deceiving, and when the ice and snow melt in the warmth of the sun, the resilient branches resume their natural positions.

I, too, am resilient, for the spirit of God is within me. God's spirit supports me as I adjust to the pressures and stresses of my life and helps me bounce back when the load becomes stressful.

Like the willow, I am flexible yet resilient. When difficult situations arise, I approach them with the peace and poise that I have gained through my times of prayer and meditation.

Flexibility and resilience keep me strong. I withstand temporary setbacks through God's eternal spirit within.

"Now we have received not the spirit of the world, but the Spirit that is from God, so that we may understand the gifts bestowed on us by God."
—1 Corinthians 2:12

Today's Message

Focus

Centered in the presence of God, I focus on making plans and carrying through with them.

Collecting my thoughts and keeping my mind focused on what is important to me, I may feel as though I am trying to round up stray sheep.

So whenever I am having a problem staying focused, I need to remember that I control my thoughts. I choose to think positive, to keep the high watch that encourages me to see the good, and to accept the good in each situation. I know good is always present, because God is always present.

Every time I turn to God, I rein in the scattered thoughts that would otherwise cause me to feel confused and discouraged. Centered in the presence of God, I am able to focus on making plans and carrying through on them. Yet I am also able to make adjustments in my plans when needed. In the process, I discover even more of the blessings God has for me.

"For you were going astray like sheep,
but now you have returned to the shepherd
and guardian of your souls."
—1 Peter 2:25

TODAY'S MESSAGE

Coping with Change

—◆—

God is with me to guide, direct, and sustain me through all life's changes.

Having made the decision to lose weight, I accept the fact that I will make changes in my lifestyle. Some of them will be easier than others. During sacred moments of prayer, I turn within to the guiding presence of God for the wisdom to know when a change is necessary and also for the strength to follow through with that change.

As with any lifestyle change, losing weight opens up new avenues of exploration for me. I give myself time to adjust to change. With God as my guide, I am able to let go of old habits and grasp new ideas. Each change becomes easier to accept, and I look for opportunities to explore new types of food, to find fun ways to exercise, and to enjoy a healthier body.

As I let go of old habits and form new ones, I understand that a thinner, healthier me is the wonderful result.

"Everything old has passed away; see, everything has become new!"
—2 Corinthians 5:17

MEDITATION

Awakened Soul

My soul is awakened to God and to the beauty of all life.

God, in this time of prayer and meditation, my soul fully awakens to You. Your spirit uplifts my thoughts to a high level of spiritual understanding, and I feel wonderfully alive!

The very essence of Your presence permeates my soul, and I radiate Your love through my thoughts and actions. I pray that all those whom I meet are aware of the peace I exude and perceive me as the awakened soul that I now am.

Thank You, God, for eyes that see the beauty of Your world, for hands that create something visible from invisible ideas, for arms and legs that give me freedom of movement.

You have entrusted me with the miracle of life, and I vow to honor my body as a sacred temple of Your spirit that it is.

"In him we live and move and have our being."
—Acts 17:28

◆ *Journal* ◆

Date: ________________________________

My weight: ___________________________

I can turn housework into exercise that benefits me as well as improves the looks of my home.

I can stretch my arms more as I vacuum or dust.
I can ________________________________

Today's Message

Enthusiasm

—◆—

I am filled with enthusiasm, for the spirit of God is active in me and through me.

Children are filled with enthusiasm. They joyously participate in their games, their activities, their very lives with a sense of freedom and abandonment. I remember that I am a child also—a child of God. That sense of freedom and abandonment lives within me, imbuing me with an enthusiasm for living.

As a child of God, I am filled with energy—the energy of Spirit. This energy carries me through the day, helps me keep a positive outlook, and enables me to do all that I have to do.

In my prayer times, I open my mind and heart to God, and I experience the joy of living in an awareness of my spirituality and of knowing that God and I are one.

Joy and enthusiasm fill my very soul and flow out into my conversations and activities. I am infused with a spirit of enthusiasm for life.

**"A new heart I will give you,
and a new spirit I will put within you."
—Ezekiel 36:26**

Today's Message

Faith

My soul and my life are enriched by my faith in God.

My faith uplifts my spirits and encourages me to listen for divine guidance in making definite decisions about an action plan of weight loss and just how to go about doing it.

Faith springs eternal as I meet the challenge of directing my energy toward greater physical well-being. I have faith that even though the results may not be dramatic in the first few weeks, I am rewarded because I know I have taken control of my life.

Praying every day and living my life with faith in God, I still may have challenges, but because I pray and because I have faith, I am able to overcome them. Life is a mystery, and I face each challenge with strength of mind and heart, for my faith in God carries me through.

With a soul enriched with faith, I can't help but remain optimistic and joy-filled.

"For the Lord gives wisdom; from his mouth come knowledge and understanding."
—Proverbs 2:6

Today's Message
Commitment

Thank You, God, for the strength and determination to be a winner.

I may not be able to recall all the times I have attempted to lose weight but have given up. So what will make this time different? This time I will succeed, because I have made a commitment to living healthier and to trusting in God to help me achieve success.

Simply saying I am committed to a diet plan is not enough. Today and every day as I spend time in prayer, I look to God for the strength. I am relying on God-power rather than my own willpower to succeed.

If I have a setback or make a wrong choice, I realize that these slips are only temporary. My success is not dependent on a single choice, but it is attained by continually renewing my determination to do what works for me.

Each time I sit down to eat, I renew that commitment to myself and to God. I give thanks for the peace of God that fills my heart and mind.

"Commit your way to the Lord; trust in him, and he will act."
—Psalms 37:5

TODAY'S MESSAGE

Never Too Late

***Turning to God in faith,
I experience a healthier, new way of living.***

There may be times in my life when I have regretted things I have said or done, times when I wanted to do more for myself or others. The good news is that it is never too late to help myself or another. It is never too late to find new ways of expressing myself and of showing others how much I care about them.

Today is a new day, a day for new beginnings, attitudes, and hopes. This is the day to overcome worries of the past and to be faith-filled and positive about the future.

As I turn to God, I am renewed with confidence. God helps me overcome any regrets I may have had or opportunities I may have let slip by and begin anew. I live in the now with faith that I am being divinely guided into a glorious new way of living, a way that brings me lasting health and happiness.

**"For whatever is born of God conquers the world.
And this is the victory that conquers
the world, our faith."
—1 John 5:4**

TODAY'S MESSAGE

Praise God!

—◆—

With praise, I give thanks to God, and I also celebrate the gift of life.

When I praise God, I feel as if the life of God within me is responding in a celebration of life. I not only have greater energy, I have a greater outlook on life. That feeling of celebration continues as I go about my day. There is a celebration that can be heard in the way that I talk and seen in the way that I walk. This is a celebration in which I unite body and soul in appreciation of God and for the gift of life:

"Thank You, God, for life that includes a mind that thinks clearly. I am learning just how creative I can be about what I eat and when I eat. I think ahead, anticipating what choices I may have and discovering more choices for healthy living.

"Thank You, God, for the gift of life. The more I respect my body, the more care and attention I give to my total health and well-being."

"Praise the Lord!
How good it is to sing praises to our God;
for he is gracious, and a song of praise is fitting."
—Psalms 147:1

Today's Message

Inspired

I open my heart and my life to divine inspiration.

The inspiration of knowing my identity as a spiritual being is a tremendously powerful motivator in helping me create a new physical image of myself.

How I look on the outside is greatly influenced by my innermost thoughts. When I allow my thoughts to be inspired by God, they motivate me in creating my experiences in life. I set myself up for success.

So I think about what I, as a spiritually inspired person, would do, and I do that. I am living according to Spirit. Inspired by God, I am not proving to others what I can do. I am showing what God can do through me when I am willing to be inspired. There is nothing more that I could ask for or receive that would be of more help to me than what God gives me each time I open my heart and my life to divine inspiration.

"Those who live according to the Spirit set their minds on the things of the Spirit."
—Romans 8:5

MEDITATION

Divinely Directed

I am divinely directed to what blesses me in realizing a leaner more agile body.

There is no reason that I have to make a decision on the spur of the moment about following a healthful eating plan. As I pray at the beginning of the day and throughout the day, I prepare myself for making right decisions. I go to God, who knows me better than I know myself:

"God, You are my wisdom in making decisions and following through on those decisions. I give You the challenge that I have had with overeating and accept that I am able to make choices that reflect a leaner, more agile body. I see myself passing up rich, high-calorie food and feeling good about doing just that. I visualize myself not only making right choices about the food I eat but also enjoying what I eat."

"Be strong and of good courage, and act. Do not be afraid or dismayed; for the Lord God, my God is with you. He will not fail you or forsake you."
—1 Chronicles 28:20

◆ *Journal* ◆

Date: ______________________________

My weight: __________________________

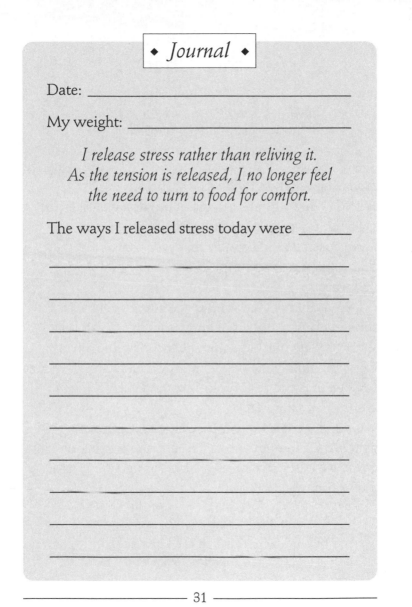

I release stress rather than reliving it.
As the tension is released, I no longer feel
the need to turn to food for comfort.

The ways I released stress today were ______

____

____

____

____

____

____

____

____

____

____

TODAY'S MESSAGE

Another Chance

—◆—

This day is another chance for me to live as a triumphant child of God.

My chances for improving my health by eating right, exercising wisely, and thinking positively are an everyday opportunity. So I go about doing all this just as I should—taking one day at a time.

Because I do, I recognize that every day is another chance for me to accomplish my goals of improving my health.

I am a child of God who is eager to give myself another chance, because I know that my Creator is ready to bless me. God strengthens me when I feel weak and uplifts me when I feel discouraged. I have the courage of a true believer in God, and such courage keeps me keeping on.

God, my constant companion, directs me to my right place and right choices even in the most confusing times. Each day is another chance for me to live as a triumphant child of God.

"The fear of others lays a snare,
but one who trusts in the Lord is secure."
—Proverbs 29:25

Today's Message

Affirm Life

My life-affirming approach to each day blesses me.

When I awaken in the morning, I have a choice to make about my day. I can choose to approach it in a negative manner or to give thanks for the blessings I am about to receive.

I choose the positive, life-affirming way. As I practice a positive approach to thinking, I am blessed physically with renewed energy. I meet my tasks with confidence, and I do what is best for myself concerning food and exercise.

Life is an adventure to be enjoyed, and I do enjoy life when I celebrate it as a glorious gift from God. How great it feels to know that God—who created each person, each creature, the Earth, the moon, the stars, and myriad universes—also created me!

I feel so blessed to be alive, alert, and enthusiastic, and I give thanks for all the blessings this day brings.

"Did I not tell you that if you believed, you would see the glory of God?"
—John 11:40

Today's Message

Look Within

Looking within my soul, I experience the unconditional love of God.

If I ever consider that I may be limited in some way, I remember that God loves me just as I am. It is important for me to love myself unconditionally as well.

I am changing the way that I look and feel physically, because this is something good I can do for myself—not because I love myself any less the way I was or am now. My spiritual nature is healthy and whole, and now is the time for me to reflect this inner glow physically and emotionally.

All that I need to accomplish this is found within me. As I look within, I find the spiritual fortitude to achieve my ideal weight.

The spirit of God infuses me with strength of soul and body. I experience a lightness of Spirit that is reflected in my appearance. I seem to stand taller and walk with greater assurance. Keeping a healthy frame of mind, I maintain a daily practice of praying and thinking positively and eating and exercising wisely.

"I have loved you with an everlasting love."
—Jeremiah 31:3

TODAY'S MESSAGE

More Than Common Sense

—◆—

God guides me to the information and people who assist me in improving and maintaining my health.

Common sense tells me that weight is more easily put on than taken off. Yet it is not always what is the easiest that is most rewarding. I am willing to make an investment in myself and my health by sticking to my weight-loss plan.

God gives me more than common sense. I rely on God to guide me in learning about health. Then I am led to informative programs, magazines, books, and to professional health care workers who contribute to that learning.

If I should digress and slip back into my old habits regarding eating and physical exercise, I try not to be hard on myself. Even though a familiar adage tells me that old habits are hard to break, I know that I can succeed with God's help and with the information and people that give me a greater understanding of how I can improve and maintain my health.

"I will restore health to you, and your wounds I will heal, says the Lord."
—Jeremiah 30:17

Today's Message

Experiencing God

As I experience God with my total being,
I know my oneness with my Creator.

One of the best things I can do for myself, for my wholeness and well-being, is to experience God with my total being. In that experience of oneness with my Creator, I let unconditional love shine in my heart, my soul, and my life.

In silence with God, I also know how it feels to be satisfied with who I am, just the way I am. Yet I understand that with God's help, I can be even better.

Living from this understanding, I am completely serene and at ease with myself and with others. I have eliminated any tendency to deal with stress by eating more. The ease I feel is reflected in the way I think and how I feel. Being stress-free, I allow my heart to function at its peak efficiency and my mind to be clear of all negativity.

The experience of experiencing God blesses me.

"As a deer longs for flowing streams,
so my soul longs for you, O God.
My soul thirsts for God, for the living God."
—Psalms 42:1–2

TODAY'S MESSAGE

New Day

I rejoice and give thanks for this new and glorious day.

As the sun peeks above the horizon and paints the sky with exquisite morning colors, I rise to greet a new day.

Yes, my body and mind are awakening and beginning the normal routine, yet I sense that more than this is happening: There is a spiritual renewal taking place in me as well. My heart rejoices for this new day, this new opportunity to be in touch with the presence of God.

I give thanks for the birds that are singing, for the laughter of children. I give thanks for being one in spirit with my Creator. With this profound sense of oneness, I can and do let go of the past and get on with this day and my plans for it.

Every day is a new day, one in which I can flow with changes and make my own. God has given me a new day, and I gratefully accept it and make the most of it.

"This is the day the Lord has made; let us rejoice and be glad in it."
—Psalms 118:24

MEDITATION

The Real Me

God created me as a unique individual; therefore, I am a creation of Spirit divine.

In a time of quiet reflection, I look past my appearance to the real me that God has created.

I close my eyes and see how God sees me—as a child born of divine love and wisdom and filled with unlimited potential.

I give thanks as God shows me that I am so much more than a physical being—I am a unique individual, a creation of Spirit divine.

Because God has shown me the truth about myself, I now feel at ease being who I am rather than hiding behind an image of what others want me to be.

I take the truth of my being with me from this time of quiet reflection: I am one of God's creations, and I have within me the potential for perfection of mind, body, and spirit. I move forward in expressing this perfection one day at a time.

"Create in me a clean heart, O God, and put a new and right spirit within me."
—Psalms 51:10

◆ *Journal* ◆

Date: ______________________________

My weight: ______________________________

I take an active role in my life.
Rather than sitting in front of the television,
I ride a stationary bike or take a walk.

I can also ______________________________

____

____

____

____

____

____

____

____

____

____

Portion sizes you'll understand:

- *A medium potato should be about the size of a computer mouse.*
- *Three ounces of meat is about the size of a cassette tape.*
- *Three ounces of grilled fish is about the size of your checkbook.*
- *One ounce of cheese is about the size of four dice.*
- *One ounce of snack foods—pretzels, etc.—equals a large handful.*

◆

SOURCE: American Dietetic Association

The Triple-Powered Approach to Health and Fitness

By Susan Smith Jones, Ph.D.

For almost 30 years, I have been teaching others how to stay healthy and fit, and I have stayed healthy and fit by living what I teach. The focus of many of the people I have worked with is to lose weight. I prefer to say lose fat, because none of us wants to lose muscle. I teach a triple-powered approach of body, mind, and spirit in achieving weight loss and fitness.

The Body

Let's begin by considering a well-rounded fitness program that includes aerobics, strength training, and stretching. Making an exercise program a top priority in life and staying committed to it unlock mental power and physical stamina and also encourage a positive outlook that makes each day more pleasurable.

Keeping Active

Aerobic exercise: Just 30 minutes of aerobic exercise 4 days a week promotes loss of body fat and decreases blood pressure, blood sugar, anxiety, depression, and insomnia. A brisk walk, hiking, cross-country skiing, and jogging are examples of aerobic activity. During aerobic exercise, fat is burned, because fat is the fuel source for the large body muscles used in such activity.

Strength training: Twice a week or more, it is important to do some type of strength training for the chest, shoulders, arms, back, and legs for at least 30 minutes each session. It's not necessary to go to a gym and use special equipment for strength training. Lifting soup cans or detergent bottles that have been emptied of detergent and then filled with water helps increase and maintain lean muscle tissue. And because lean muscle tissue is more metabolically active than fat, the body with more lean muscle burns more calories.

Flexibility: Now we add flexibility exercise. Gentle stretching or yoga along with aerobic exercise and strength training complete a program that reduces bone loss, maintains strength and muscle mass, and keeps our energy levels revved.

Nutrition and Fiber

The main emphasis with nutrition is on whole foods, which means eating foods as close to the way nature made them as possible. Every time food is cooked—whether by baking, frying, steaming, or microwaving—it loses some of its nutritional value and fiber content.

Nutrients: The antioxidants—such as vitamins C and E, and various carotenoids and flavonoids—in fresh, raw

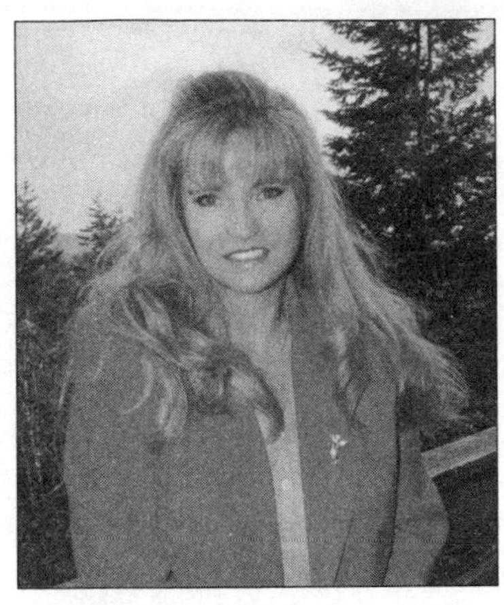

fruits and vegetables neutralize free radicals so that they lose their destructive power over cells. Eating an antioxidant-rich diet bolsters our protection from all types of disease. I recommend eating at least 5 servings of fruits and vegetables a day, selecting produce that is rich and diverse in color. Antioxidants are also the pigments that give produce a red, yellow, green, or orange color.

Fiber: The soluble fiber in oat bran, legumes, beans, peas, and lentils helps stabilize the blood-sugar level and decrease the level of cholesterol in the body. Insoluble fiber, which is found in fruits and vegetables, increases the bulk in the digestive system so that we feel full more quickly and longer.

Helpful Tips

Water: Drinking enough water is crucial to weight loss. In addition to transporting vital nutrients, water regulates body temperature, eases digestion, lubricates joints, helps eliminate waste, and keeps the skin healthy, youthful, and attractive. A shortage of water results in excess water weight, because the body has stored water outside of the cells, creating that heavy, bloated feeling.

Drinking at least eight glasses of water a day helps us achieve and maintain a healthy weight. Water is calorie-free, suppresses the appetite, and helps metabolize fat. Initially, we might spend more time in the bathroom, but the body adapts within a day or two.

Sleep: I believe there is nothing more restorative for the body, with the exception of meditation, than getting enough sleep. I know from my own life that sleep depravation causes irritability and impatience. Sleep is one of the most important components of living a balanced life.

When we reach those deep levels of sleep—the delta level—the body releases, among other things, the human growth hormone, which revitalizes and renews the body and helps the body build lean muscle. Restful sleep also lowers the level of stress hormones that have accumulated during the day.

Breakfast: Eating breakfast is important, because breaking a fast by eating breakfast stokes our metabolism. Skipping breakfast is an alert to the body, which in all its wisdom decides: "Whoa! I'm not getting any breakfast! I'd better hold on to every calorie I get, because I'm not sure when I'm going to get my next meal!"

Smaller meals but more of them: When weight loss is a goal, it's better to eat five or six small meals during the day, rather than one or two large meals. The same amount of total calories may be taken in, yet eating more food than the body can handle at one time can actually deposit more fat in the body. Eating five or six smaller meals during the day keeps the metabolism revved and burns more fat.

The Mind

The second factor in the triple-powered approach to health and fitness is the mind. In order to reduce stress and live a more balanced life, we use the formative power of our thoughts to help us create our experiences in life.

Positive thinking: Number one is the focus of our thoughts, so that what we continually think about, we bring about in our life. So we begin with our thoughts and attention on only those things that we want to bring into our life. We then visualize the end result.

I have led guided meditations in which people see themselves in their minds' eyes, living the lifestyle they want to live, looking how they want to look. As they visualize, I encourage them to experience feelings of joy and thanksgiving as if their visions were their current realities. Changing our inner thoughts, we change our outer lives.

Affirmations: Using daily affirmations is a powerful way to begin the day. I have read *Daily Word* magazine for over 25 years. I carry *Daily Word* and affirmation cards with me and affirm how I want to be and live. Working with the idea of weight loss, I might affirm: *I am naturally slender and fit and healthy and enthusiastic about life* or *I always make healthy food and fitness choices* or *I love to work out!* I keep affirmations near me—at my desk, on my bathroom mirror, and next to my bed. I fill my mind with thoughts that help me create my day.

The Spirit

We apply the third approach as we disconnect from the outer world and reconnect with God's spirit within us so that we are recharged with love, power, and vitality. I find it helpful to bookend my day, once in the morning and once in the evening, with prayer and meditation.

Whenever we turn within, we realize that we are never alone in anything we are trying to accomplish. We act in a partnership of cocreating our life with God.

Meditation: As we daily reconnect with God in quiet moments of meditation, we live from an awareness of God and make choices that enhance our well-being throughout the day. I meditate while spending time in nature. After a hike in the crisp morning air, I realize that whatever problems and challenges I thought I had at the beginning of the hike are usually dissolved. Or at least I am able to see them from a higher vantage point or perspective at the end of the hike. I have not only been physically active, I have also fed my soul.

When we reconnect with the divine power within us, we no longer feel empty. We are filled spiritually and no longer look for things outside ourselves, such as drugs, alcohol, work, overeating, shopping, or gambling to fulfill us. We are complete within.

Breathing: Breath is a part of our spiritual awareness. So in making our health a top priority, we make breathing right a top priority. Taking a 2-minute break every hour on the hour, we make a commitment to consciously breathe slowly and deeply, with our spine straight. Not only do we more fully oxygenate our body, which makes our body more efficiently burn fat as a fuel source, but we calm ourselves so that we relax. From this relaxed state of being, we remain stress-free and view life with a positive perspective.

The Miraculous Body

God has given us this incredible gift of a miraculous body, and one of the gifts that we can give back to God is to take good care of ourselves. When we release the emotional baggage that we have been carrying with us and begin treating ourselves with respect and kindness, we discover that our behavior and our lives mirror how good we feel about ourselves.

Ben Franklin once said that whatever a person does for 21 days will make or break a habit. That's good advice. Just think: In 21 days, whether you decide to agree with yourself to work out or eat healthier or get enough sleep or establish all of these good habits, you will be leaner, healthier, and more fit. I know you can do it!

Today's Message

I Can

Through the power of the indwelling presence of God, I am successful.

Although I have made a personal commitment to follow a weight-loss program, there may be times when I wonder if I can carry out this commitment. If I have doubt or concern, I only have to look within to find inner strength. As I search within my soul, I realize that I can do anything I set my mind and heart on, for the power of God supports me.

God's presence within—that perfect potential within me—enables me to do all things. Through my awareness of God, I can and do accomplish my aims. I have the strength, the stamina, the motivation to be successful in attaining my ideal weight.

As I relax and trust the power of God within me, I am certain that I can keep my commitment and that I will see results. The certainty of God's presence is my constant inspiration.

"Jesus said to them, 'Do you believe that I am able to do this? . . . According to your faith let it be done to you.'"
—Matthew 9:28–29

TODAY'S MESSAGE

I Am Loved and Loving

God loves me, and I am loving.

God loves me, and I do all that I can to honor and cherish myself as a beloved creation of God.

As I affirm *God loves me* several times a day, I am strengthened physically, emotionally, and spiritually. I consider, "How shall I treat a beloved creation of God?" The answer is, "With love": "Love is patient and kind . . . rejoices in the right. Love is not irritable or resentful." (1 Cor. 13:4)

So I am patient and kind with myself. I rejoice over my accomplishments. I am loving, so I treat others as God's beloved creations. I am patient and kind with them also, rejoicing in their achievements.

God loves me is an affirmation that lifts me up and keeps me motivated. I complete the circle of love by being loving. Yes, God loves me, and I am loving.

**"For the mountains may depart and the hills be removed,
but my steadfast love shall not depart from you,
and my covenant of peace shall not be removed,
says the Lord, who has compassion on you."
—Isaiah 54:10**

Today's Message

Perception

—◆—

I am a divine creation—unchanging in spirit but changeable in form.

Unkind jokes or comments about my weight by others may cause me to feel less than happy about my appearance, but only if I let them. The opinions and words of others are powerless against my belief that I am perfect and whole in the sight of God.

Others might question why I would want to go on a diet or change the way I look if I feel I am perfect. I would tell them: "I know that because I am divinely created, I have a spiritual perfection. If my outer appearance needs some improvement, God will guide me in what to do and how to do it. The physical me is changeable, but Spirit within me is constant and unchanging perfection."

I want to keep my thoughts of myself in line with my perception of how God must surely see me—perfect in spirit and a work in progress physically. I am unique, created in and sustained by divine love.

"By the grace of God I am what I am,
and his grace toward me has not been in vain."
—1 Corinthians 15:10

Today's Message

Precious Light

—◆—

Reflecting the light of God within, I experience the fullness of joy.

A diamond has many facets that, when they reflect the light, can dazzle the eye and inspire awe in the beholder. Today I choose to see my life as a multi-faceted diamond that reflects the light of God.

When I consider my life from this perspective, I understand that each new day offers me experiences through which I can allow God's light to radiate from me as joy on my journey through life. I approach each opportunity with feelings of anticipation and enthusiasm, for I know that I have the precious light of God's wisdom to guide me.

If a facet of my life seems to challenge me, I know that the light of God will shine from within to show me how to make greater progress and to do it with courage and grace. With God's light, I have confidence and poise, and in this awareness, a deep feeling of joy rises up to soothe me.

"Teach us to count our days that we may gain a wise heart."
—Psalms 90:12

Today's Message
Breakthrough

Each breakthrough to a new level of accomplishment encourages me to keep trying.

In my prayer time, I have learned to be patient and wait for the guidance I desire and the answers I seek. I do all that I know to do and then wait on God. When the guidance or answer comes, I feel a joy and lightness of spirit that make me feel as if I could soar.

I expect the same uplifting feeling as I look for and discover a successful way to lose weight. I may try several diet plans, but when I find one that I am comfortable with and works for me, I will know this is the one for me to follow.

I break free from old habits and rise above circumstances that would hinder my progress. Just as each answered prayer renews my faith, each breakthrough to a new level of accomplishment encourages me to keep trying.

**"They will break through and pass the gate,
going out by it. Their king will pass on before them,
the Lord at their head."
—Micah 2:13**

TODAY'S MESSAGE

Achievement

My greatest achievement is including more time in my day for communion with God.

Maybe I have never thought about less ever being a greater achievement than more. Certainly less weight is near the top of my wish list. However, maybe less of some things will help me achieve this.

Reducing my food intake is the first thing that comes to mind. What if I found less to complain about in general? Then I would discover more for which I am thankful. That thankfulness is very satisfying.

Less time watching television will give me more time to pray and meditate. Prayer and meditation are ways that I tap into the very presence of God within me. The more of God I include in my day, the less frustration I experience. The less frustration I feel, the more in control of my life I can be.

Doing less of some things will give me more time to do what fortifies me, such as communing with God so that I am prepared to achieve.

"Now to him who by the power at work within us is able to accomplish abundantly far more than all we can ask or imagine, to him be glory."
—Ephesians 3:20–21

MEDITATION
Affirmations

My affirmations are positive statements of truth that I use to claim my good.

The positive affirmations I speak bring about greater good in me and through me. So I take this affirmation into my meditation: *I am a wonderfully constructed creation of the Creator of all life.*

With my eyes closed, I repeat this affirmation and let the truth of it resonate within me: *I am a wonderfully constructed creation of the Creator of all life.*

How could I think of myself or any other creation of God as anything less than wonderful? The question stirs a response within the depths of my soul that rises up though me, cleansing me of any feelings of rejection or disappointment. I feel good emotionally and physically as I linger in the warm glow of the realization of who I am. Yes, I am ready to live as the wonderfully constructed creation of the Creator of all life that I am.

"So shall my word be that goes out from my mouth; it shall not return to me empty, but it shall accomplish that which I purpose, and succeed in the thing for which I sent it."
—Isaiah 55:11

◆ *Journal* ◆

Date: ________________________________

My weight: ____________________________

A good weight-loss plan takes careful planning of meals and activities.

Today I plan to __________________________

____

____

____

____

____

____

____

____

____

____

Today's Message

Cherished Moments

—◆—

I give thanks for cherished moments, for they are gifts from God.

This day cannot be relived, so I do not waste a moment of it. I live to the fullest by recognizing each day as a treasure chest of cherished moments.

In order to enjoy my day, I need the energy that keeps me alert and enthusiastic. With exercise and nutritious foods, I can boost my energy level, which enables me to live my day fully and completely.

Today holds the promise of cherished moments—golden times with special people and of fulfilling experiences. God's glory is constantly being revealed to me, and I am grateful that I am a part of that glory. I am also grateful that I can use my time, my talents, and my love to be a source of cherished moments for others. Together we give and receive from the presence of God within us so that we continue building cherished moments that fill our lives with meaning and purpose.

I give thanks for the gift of each moment.

"How much better to get wisdom than gold! To get understanding is to be chosen rather than silver." —Proverbs 16:16

Today's Message
Expectations

My expectations are a preview of the new me that is emerging.

My expectations of weight loss are not based solely on the kind and amount of food I eat or the intensity and frequency of my exercise. My expectations of a new slimmer, more energetic, and healthier me are based on what the power of the Almighty can do through me.

Because there is no limit to what God can do, I never limit my thoughts of what God can do through *me*. I expect God to strengthen me if I feel weak—physically or emotionally. I expect God to guide me if I am confused. I expect God to heal me of all feelings of unworthiness or inadequacy.

I have great expectations of myself also: I expect that I will listen, learn, and act on the guidance of God. My expectations are a preview of a new me that is emerging. I see myself as I can and will be as I continue to keep my expectations positive and positively on what God can do through me.

"See, the former things have come to pass, and new things I now declare; before they spring forth, I tell you of them."
—Isaiah 42:9

TODAY'S MESSAGE

Encouragement

Yes, God, I am encouraged and ready to succeed!

Old habits may seem to beckon to me at every turn, but I am strong, because my positive words energize me. They are a spark of truth that rejuvenates me. My body responds to the encouraging words that I speak.

I would never want to hold myself back by thinking that I am limited in some way. I am so much more than a physical being—I am spiritual perfection! I am energized, and the life of God-life within uplifts me and inspires me to continue on. I am alive with the life of God!

If an obstacle seems to stand in my way, I know I can overcome it. If I feel discouraged because I have a long way to go before I reach my weight-loss goal, I know that, given my time and my dedication, the way grows shorter each day.

All the while, God encourages and strengthens me so that I will succeed!

"Not that I have already obtained this or have already reached the goal; but I press on to make it my own."
—Philippians 3:12

Today's Message

Self-Esteem

My positive self-esteem emerges from my inner spiritual nature.

A positive self-image is important to me, for it is reflected in every thought I think and every action I take. When I feel good about who I am, then I will feel good about whatever I am doing as well. Such self-esteem emerges whenever I have a realization of my inner spiritual nature.

For instance, whether I am interacting with people for the first time or after many times, I have a confidence that shows on my face and can be heard in the tone of my voice. I am comfortable working with people, and I also put them at ease.

Having positive people around me is important in maintaining my own self-esteem. I feel good when I have a healthy self-confidence, so I naturally want to surround myself with those who have a positive outlook as well. We encourage one another to know that we are special to God and to one another.

"Our inner nature is being renewed day by day."
—2 Corinthians 4:16

TODAY'S MESSAGE

Learning

I am learning more about myself each day, and I give thanks to God for my capacity to learn.

Life is a spiritual journey, and every day I am learning something new.

I am learning about what is good for me: what foods give a boost to my overall health and what exercises give me the best workout. I am also learning about my emotions: how I can achieve greater peace of mind. I am learning about my spirituality: how to more deeply experience the presence of God. As I learn, I nourish my body, nurture my mind, and enrich my soul.

The most important detail I can know about myself is that I am a spiritual being, walking a spiritual path with God. With each step I take, I remind myself that I am learning and growing.

I give thanks to God today for my capacity to learn. With each lesson, I gain a greater understanding of my true self and of my ability to accomplish whatever I set out to accomplish—and even more.

"Take my yoke upon you,
and learn from me."
—Matthew 11:29

TODAY'S MESSAGE

Recharged

I am recharged and ready for this day!

Food and rest, exercise and sleep recharge me mentally and physically. Each has a time and a space to fill in my day. Hopefully, I will have 8 hours of sleep, give both my body and mind a good workout, and eat nutritious meals in any 24-hour period. I will take a couple of breaks and have a couple of snacks too.

Yet, I also need to experience a spiritual energy. As I tap into the sacred center of my soul and commune with God, I fairly tingle with an awareness of the power within me. I am recharged with a sense of my own sacredness and a purpose to fulfill today.

I may spend time paying bills or studying for a test. When I feel stuck or bored—instead of searching in the refrigerator for something to eat—I meditate for 10 minutes or take a brisk walk. Fresh inspiration and fresh air revive me so that I remain ready for this day.

"But those who wait for the Lord shall renew their strength, they shall mount up with wings like eagles, they shall run and not be weary, they shall walk and not faint."
—Isaiah 40:31

MEDITATION

Counting My Blessings

I thank God every day for my blessings.

In a time of communication with God, I feel a sacred stirring within my soul:

"God, I open the way to a multitude of wondrous blessings when I allow You to be God in my life. Because I realize that You are so much more than I can ever comprehend, I release any preconceived ideas of how I think You will bless me. I no longer limit my blessings in any way.

"The blessings I have received in the past have been momentous, such as the miraculous healing—of myself or someone I love. Or the blessing may be a subtle reminder of Your wonder, such as witnessing a peaceful valley from a mountaintop or receiving a warm embrace from a loved one. In whatever form they may take, I count my blessings and give thanks to You."

**"His divine power has given us everything needed for life and godliness, through the knowledge of him who called us by his own glory and goodness."
—2 Peter 1:3–4**

◆ *Journal* ◆

Date: ______________________________

My weight: __________________________

I am celebrating
the little successes that I
have accomplished.

I pat myself on the back for ______________

____

____

____

____

____

____

____

____

____

____

TODAY'S MESSAGE

Sense of Humor

Laughter is music from God that reverberates throughout my being.

My entire body responds to my laughter. When I laugh, my lungs take in more oxygen and my heart beats stronger. My body is releasing any tension and stress, and I feel so alive. Laughter is music from God that reverberates throughout my spirit, mind, and body.

I welcome the joy of laughter and humor into my day. My outlook on life is always brighter when I maintain a sense of humor. Rather than focusing on negative situations, I find that there is something humorous about them.

I keep a positive attitude by remembering to laugh at myself. I lighten up so that I am not critical of the way I look or how close I am following my diet. Any weight I may have gained will not be as quick to come off as it was to put on, but laughter will make my way easier.

I look forward to the rest of my day and to each chance to laugh again.

"The joy of the Lord is your strength."
—Nehemiah 8:10

Today's Message

God Is My Help

God is my help in all and through all.

My greatest desire is to be one with the presence of God. Because I put God first, all that I experience is blessed with the enrichment of my spiritual awareness. I realize that what may seem like such a challenge is a call for me to better myself.

There is nothing beyond God's ability to heal or renew. If I need greater strength of mind or body, I affirm and reaffirm that God is my strength.

During those times when I feel discouraged about my weight loss or current weight, I call on God for help. God lifts me higher than I ever imagined possible.

I matter to God, and God is my help in all and through all. In a moment of reflection, I encourage myself: "I am one of God's creations. God does not create anything less than what is perfect in spirit. I let this perfection of spirit live out through me so that I am living as God created me to live."

"Surely God is my salvation; I will trust, and will not be afraid."
—Isaiah 12:2

Today's Message

Move Forward

◆

With God as my guide, I move forward to a happier, healthier lifestyle.

I have learned from experience how to lose weight. Yet I am still making positive changes in my lifestyle, so I don't let looking back at where I have been cause me to lose sight of where I am going.

I trust God to help me let go of what is not bringing about good results and to show me a new, better way. With each experience cheering me on, I keep moving toward my desired weight.

It helps me to compare this process to one I would use to cross a creek: Moving from one stepping-stone or lost pound—no matter how small it may seem—to another, I make progress.

If ever I feel as if I am stuck in the middle of that creek or process, I will need encouragement so that I won't turn back. I look to God to direct me so that I continue to move forward. In sacred moments of prayer, I receive the inspiration and encouragement to move on.

"Forgetting what lies behind and straining forward to what lies ahead, I press on toward the goal."
—Philippians 3:13–14

Today's Message

Optimistic

I am optimistic!

Can I picture myself wearing a size smaller pair of slacks in a few months? Of course, I can. Now can I believe that I can make this picture a reality? Yes, I am optimistic, and my optimism is an incentive to me. I am both optimistic and motivated.

What more do I need to complete this new picture of me? It requires some effort on my part and the passing of time. Confidence in myself will help. Yet my faith in God to be my ever-present source of inspiration and understanding, courage and determination is essential.

A spark of optimism leads me on in making the picture of the improved and happier me. And when more than optimism, confidence, and motivation are needed, God is here with me to give me more. God blesses me far above and beyond anything I can picture for myself. I believe in God with all my heart and soul.

"I believe that I shall see the goodness of the Lord in the land of the living."
—Psalms 27:13

Today's Message

Heart Blessing

My commitment to pray, eat right, and exercise blesses my heart.

Without me ever having to tell my heart what to do, it pumps steadily, supplying my body with the life-giving nourishment it needs to sustain and renew itself.

The more overweight I am, however, the harder my heart has to work. So I remember to bless my heart in my prayers and to eat nourishing foods in the proper amounts so that I keep my weight within a healthy range. I then help my heart continue its vital work.

As I walk or jog to stimulate my circulation, I silently bless my heart with prayer:

"Dear God, thank You for the fascinating, intricate workings of my body and especially of my heart. I appreciate the strength that my heart has as it pumps steadily, and I do not take it for granted. Rather, I do what I can to keep it healthy and strong. Thank You, God, for my healthy heart."

**"If we live by the Spirit,
let us also be guided by the Spirit."
—Galatians 5:25**

Today's Message

Forgiving Myself

Letting God's love guide me,
I forgive myself and begin a fresh start.

An important goal for me right now is to let go of the past and go on with my life. And one thing that will help me do this is to forgive myself for any past action that may have kept me from expressing my true self, my divine nature.

I know that by forgiving myself, I am doing what is essential for me to do in order to make progress in life. The still, small voice of God's spirit within tells me that by forgiving myself, I will begin to heal past hurts and make a fresh start.

Quiet times of prayer help me do this, for in prayer I connect—at a deep soul level—with the infinite love of God. God's love is powerful, yet gentle, and it guides me in seeing myself as God sees me—with love and compassion. I gently remind myself to leave past decisions where they belong—in the past. Letting God's love guide me, I make wise choices.

"Whenever you stand praying, forgive."
—Mark 11:25

Meditation

Inner Reality

Because God's spirit resides within me, I have an inner divine reality.

In a quiet, secluded place, I let my thoughts move past the form and shape that identifies me physically to my inner reality that identifies me spiritually.

My spiritual identity is eternal divine life in expression. Divine life is expressing through my mind and body whether I realize it or not. But in meditation, I put all activities and thoughts aside and move into a full realization of my own sacredness.

In this moment, I know that God's spirit resides within me and all around me. My mind and body cannot shape or form Spirit, but Spirit can help me shape and reform my body, for God is all power and wisdom. Now I know that during times that some craving for more is pushing me toward overindulgence, I can release the power and wisdom of my inner reality and say, "No!"

"To them God chose to make known how great among the Gentiles are the riches of the glory of this mystery, which is Christ in you, the hope of glory."
—Colossians 1:27

◆ *Journal* ◆

Date: ____________________

My weight: ____________________

I forgive myself for my mistakes
and others for any actions that may have hurt me.
Feelings of animosity are replaced with ones
of love and acceptance.

I forgive ____________________

____

____

____

____

____

____

____

____

____

TODAY'S MESSAGE
In Control

I take the initiative and act on my God-given ability to take control of my weight.

If I think that my weight is out of control, I need to sit down and have a talk with myself. I know the choices to make about the way I eat and exercise, and when I carry through with them, I am in control!

My dress size may never be a single digit number, but I can be a healthier, more energetic person by setting my weight goal at what is realistic for me.

I think nothing of taking the initiative to control the thermostat in my home and the water temperature of my shower or bath. I also take the initiative to be in control of my weight.

God has given me the ability to reason and to plan, to be creative and wise. The more I use these abilities, the stronger they are and easier to use. By taking control, I make a great investment in my physical and emotional health.

"What are human beings that you are mindful of them, or mortals, that you care for them? You have made them for a little while lower than the angels; you have crowned them with glory and honor."
—Hebrews 2:6–7

Today's Message

Divine Appointment

—◆—

I am showing up for all my divine appointments today.

Why is it that on a day that I try so hard to accomplish something, I seem to meet with all kinds of detours and obstacles? Then, when I am exerting the least amount of effort in arranging my life, my day goes so smoothly?

I believe the smooth days are divine appointment days—when I have put myself in the flow of a divine plan and I am cooperating with God in all that I do. Because I have ceased to struggle and I have tuned in to my divine appointments, I show up for them. I am working with God to accomplish small and great tasks.

I eat right and I sleep well. I think clearly and I plan wisely. I have patience with myself and others. Knowing that I am on the right track, I move steadily forward, giving thanks to God for my divine appointment day. I accept and follow through with the opportunities this day presents to me.

**"For everything there is a season,
and a time for every matter under heaven."
—Ecclesiastes 3:1**

TODAY'S MESSAGE

Full Life

God has given me a spirit, mind, and body; I can and do live a full life.

Knowing that the thoughts I hold in mind shape my experiences is a truth that helps shape my day and me.

So thinking about and giving thanks that I am fulfilled shifts my focus and helps me to be successful. I live a full life because God has created me whole—with a spirit, mind, and body. When my body seems to be demanding more fuel, I think about what kind and amount of food I need for energy: More than likely, a fresh piece of fruit will give me a boost of energy with no extra calories to be stored. Maybe what my body needs is exercise, not food. So I take a walk around my neighborhood or in the park. I notice the fullness of life around me—people, trees, flowers, and birds.

And during those times I cannot seem to think my way to a solution, I pray. Prayer satisfies my soul, and a satisfied soul conveys the joy of living a full life to both mind and body.

"You show me the path of life. In your presence there is fullness of joy; in your right hand are pleasures forevermore."
—Psalms 16:11

Today's Message

A Time and Place

I pray for loved ones, knowing that God will bless them in perfect and timely ways.

I support others with my positive thoughts when they are trying to lose weight. Because there is a right time and place for me to offer my help, I realize that I may not need to say or do anything more than to pray for them and know that whatever they need will be provided.

Even though I may have the best interests of others at heart, past experiences have shown that sometimes conversations about eating in healthy ways or keeping fit may not fall on receptive ears. My enthusiasm about healthy eating patterns and fitness habits has a positive effect on my own well-being. However, I maintain a sensitivity to the physical and emotional needs of friends and family members by curbing that zeal and redirecting it into my prayer times.

I enfold my family and friends in thoughts of strength, wisdom, life, and love, knowing that in God's tender care, they will be blessed.

"Let all that you do be done in love."
—1 Corinthians 16:14

Today's Message

Rhythm of Life

I am one with the rhythm of life that is resounding throughout all creation.

There is a vital rhythm of life resounding within all of God's creation. This divine rhythm resonates in the ebb and flow of the tides and in the voices of loved ones.

There is a rhythm of life within me as well. This rhythm is God-life moving in and through me. I experience it in the steady beat of my heart as it rests and contracts, in the rise and fall of my lungs as I breathe, and in the flow of my life's blood as it courses through my arteries and veins.

I am one with the rhythm of life—divine life within and surrounding me that renews me in mind and body. With each breath I take, with each beat of my heart, I am aware of the powerful rhythm of life that fills me and energizes me. Aware that I am a divine creation, I give thanks for the vital rhythm of God-life that is resounding in me and throughout all creation.

"Out of the believer's heart shall flow rivers of living water."
—John 7:38

Today's Message

New Doors

—◆—

God opens new doors of blessings to me, and I eagerly go forth through them.

I have often heard that when one door closes, God opens another one, and I believe this is true. Reflecting on my life, I recognize the many times that God led me to new doors that were open to blessings that were mine as a part of my divine heritage from my Creator.

Each day is one in which I can celebrate the gift of life and give thanks for new blessings. I myself or others may not consider me perfect, and, thank God, I do not have to be! But today is a new day in which I can do my best in continuing to improve myself and to be the best person I know how to be.

I welcome the chance to prove what God can do through me. So with an awareness of God, I let go of any illusion of limitation and eagerly enter through new doors to accept my blessings.

"By paths they have not known
I will guide them.
I will turn the darkness before them into light,
the rough places into level ground."
—Isaiah 42:16

Meditation
Shelter of Love

In silence with God,
I retreat to a shelter of love.

My mind is a gateway that leads to a place of love and peace. The keys that open that gate are my prayers and my quiet talks with God.

Settling into my chair, I close my eyes and breathe deeply and evenly. As I focus on my breathing, I feel tension being replaced with a sense of peace and well-being.

I have entered through a gateway into a divine realm where God waits for me. In this quiet refuge, I am surrounded by God's pure, unconditional love.

Love is always there, because God is always there. I leave this place secure in the knowledge that I can always turn to God, the infinite source of love, and be renewed with strength and peace that continually sustain me.

"I am convinced that neither death, nor life,
nor angels, nor rulers, nor things present,
nor things to come, nor powers, nor height,
nor depth, nor anything else in creation, will be able
to separate us from the love of God."
—Romans 8:38–39

◆ *Journal* ◆

Date: ______________________________

My weight: __________________________

I welcome new doors
of opportunity that God
opens before me.

My new opportunities may include ________

____

____

____

____

____

____

____

____

____

____

Drink plenty of water before, during, and after walking, especially when it's hot or humid. If you're going to walk in the heat for an hour, drink water at least 15 minutes before you go out and every 15 minutes during your walk. (If you walk longer than an hour, drink a carbohydrate and salt replacement drink, like Gatorade.) Don't wait until you feel thirsty to drink. On long walks, carry water.

◆

Source: Prevention's Complete Book of Walking
by Maggie Spilner

Achieving Wholeness of Spirit, Mind, and Body

By Edie Hand

Over the past 20 years, I have had various occurrences of cancer, and I am happy to say that I am a cancer survivor. In my 20s, I was diagnosed with cancer of the uterus. Later I had a kidney removed because of cancer. Then about 3 years ago, I learned that I had breast cancer. Thanks to my regular checkups, the doctors discovered the cancer at an early stage and removed it surgically with a lumpectomy.

In between my bouts with cancer, my weight would yo-yo: I was overweight, back to normal, and a few months later I might be 25 pounds overweight. Having a career in entertainment and public speaking, I was concerned about my weight. Speaking in front of an audience and performing on my television show, I was conscious of my weight and struggled to control it.

I finally came to an understanding that what I really needed was to do much more than control my weight; I needed to achieve wholeness—a balance of spirit, mind, and body. Through prayer, I sought God's help in achieving this balance. As I prayed, I gained strength, confidence, and knowledge that helped me lose weight and keep it off. I started making better choices about the food

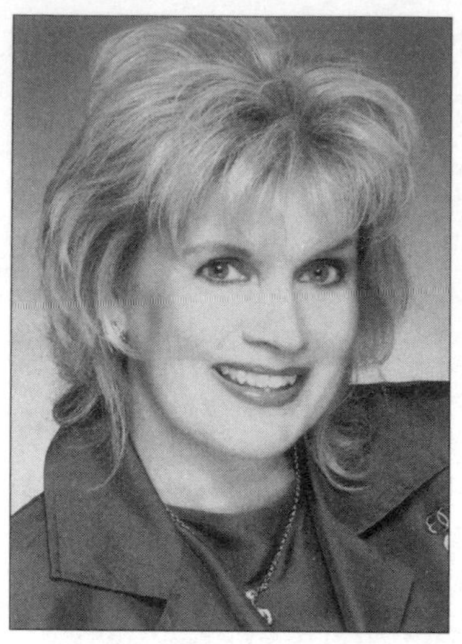

I ate, and I learned how to cook lighter—reducing my intake of fat. I became more aware of the calories that I was taking in and reduced the amount. I also started a simple exercise program and got more rest. For many years I had sustained myself on a maximum of 5 hours of sleep per night. That simply was not enough.

I realized that just as there are important ingredients in a recipe, there are also important ingredients to life. I could be on a diet program, but if I didn't have a positive attitude and make the right choices about all aspects of my life, I was just applying a temporary fix.

When I was growing up, my days were filled with good food and good people. The family picnics held at my grandparents' house were fun times that included aunts, uncles, and cousins. My cousin Elvis Presley and my great-aunt Minnie, Elvis's grandmother, shared in some of those good times of traditional Southern food and family fun.

Now that I am an adult, I know I need the discipline of planning my meals so that I eat nutritious foods in the right amounts. I take the time to shop selectively, having my menu with me as I look for the leanest meats. I cook "lighter" by using canola oil. These are the types of healthy decisions that are important to make every day in planning meals no matter what my schedule.

In the past when I was on the road for several weeks, I would gain 10 to 15 pounds. Once I was home, I would starve myself, trying to lose the weight as quickly as possible. This would only lead to another unpleasant development: painful migraine headaches. I have learned that less fat and more protein in my diet, accompanied by exercise, meant fewer migraines.

Keeping a positive attitude toward weight control and the complexities of life is not always easy. When I feel my attitude sinking, I shut my thoughts down and listen to what God is telling me. I want and need answers, so I ask for them in prayer. Those answers come to me in different ways, and they help to strengthen me and build my confidence.

Faith in God has carried me through some dark hours, but although my life has changed, my faith has deepened. Two of my beloved brothers died young, and Terry, my surviving brother, is living with a brain aneurism that is slowly taking away all of his motor skills. Life is precious, and I turn to God for guidance to be where I need to be and do what I need to do to help Terry and the rest of my family. When Terry's health began to decline, I felt as if I was being pulled down into the depths of despair. My faith has grown since that time, and now, when I am with Terry, I am focused on him—helping him and being strong for him. Each time I leave him, I pray a prayer of faith and turn him over to God.

I practice the same letting go and letting God concerning my finances, my health, and my diet. No one is going to fix things for me. There is no magic wand that I can wave, but what I can do is turn to God for strength and comfort.

I have been blessed with wonderful friends who have stood by my side through all of my challenges. I try to keep people around me who have a positive attitude. One thing I have learned is to respond to people from the spirit of God within me, not to react to them by mirroring their emotions. For example, if someone seems angry or upset, I do not react to that anger by being angry or upset myself. I take a moment to breathe deeply, focus on God, and respond in a positive way. In that moment, I communicate with God so that I am able to be a peacekeeper.

I have learned to look at my finances in a positive way also. I went through a divorce 12 years ago, and I had changes to deal with that affected me both emotionally and financially. I learned how to budget and how to keep a healthy balance in my finances by including God in all my decisions. With God's help, I began to set goals for my short-term needs, and then I focused on the long-term. By keeping focused on God and on my goals rather than my finances, I found that the money would come. Faith and simple adjustments have helped me through the stresses of life.

Simple things like morning stretches and walking have changed my life. When I get up in the morning, I have a glass of orange juice and do five basic stretching exercises that loosen my lower back, my arms, and my legs. I feel that this kick-starts my metabolism and gives me energy throughout the day. My goal is to walk every day or at least to walk every other day. Over time I have built up my endurance so that I can walk 2 to 3 miles at a brisk pace. As I walk, I also swing my arms and keep my back erect, which I believe relieves me of fluid retention.

In the first 6 weeks of making these simple changes in my life—reducing fat and calories, cooking light, walking more and drinking 8 to 10 glasses of water a day—I lost 10 pounds. It was during this time that I realized that my diet and exercise benefited me physically, my positive attitude refreshed me mentally and emotionally, and my faith nourished me spiritually. I felt that I was forming a more complete and balanced life.

If I get up in the morning and feel more tired than usual, I know that I need to exercise that day and include a little more protein in my diet. I have tried a lot of fad diets in my life during my yo-yo years, but never before have I experienced the positive results and peace of mind that I do now.

I have learned from my own experiences, not only about the basics of diet and exercise, but about balance for my whole self—spirit, mind, and body. I share my experiences with groups and organizations in seminars entitled *Attitude for Life*.

In 2001, I was asked by the makers of Mazola canola oil to be their spokesperson on a 12-city tour. On this tour, I shared recipes from my book, *Recipes for Life,* and conducted cooking demonstrations at the Mazola Canola "Good to Know Ya" van, a 20-foot mobile kitchen designed to resemble a traditional country home with a white picket fence, a front porch, and rocking chairs. As I toured with *Southern Living Cooking Schools* and attended various fairs and festivals across the South, I have had the opportunity to make new friends and to share my experiences with them.

Experiences in life led me to understand that I needed to achieve wholeness—a balance of spirit, mind, and body. I now feel whole and well—physically, emotionally, and spiritually—and I am grateful that this balance continues to open new doors of opportunity in my life.

TODAY'S MESSAGE

All Things Are Possible

With God's help, all things are possible for me and are being revealed to me.

A small seed is filled with endless possibilities. This tiny form of nature has the innate capacity to be transformed into a vibrant, exquisite flower.

I, too, am filled with endless possibilities, and I am being transformed every day. Each day, I am becoming more comfortable with myself, more attuned to what my body needs, more peaceful in mind and heart. My transformation is spiritual as well, for I am spending time with God in quiet contemplation and prayer.

What a glorious transformation I am experiencing, and what endless possibilities lie before me! Like the small seed, I am becoming all that I can become and more. I believe that with God's help all things are possible, and I believe that great possibilities are being revealed to me now.

"For truly I tell you, if you have faith the size of a mustard seed, you will say to this mountain, 'Move from here to there,' and it will move; and nothing will be impossible for you."
—Matthew 17:20

TODAY'S MESSAGE

Stream of Life

I am moving on in life and making progress.

How do I handle stress? Thinking and eating, resting and exercising in ways that build and maintain my physical and emotional well-being relieve me of stress. I move on with life instead of becoming stuck thinking about why something happened to me.

For instance, if I gained instead of lost weight this past week, I won't waste time agonizing over the fact that I did have a weight gain. Just as life moves on, I also move on—with my program—knowing that I will do better.

It is good to know if anything I have done or not done has caused me to gain weight, such as not keeping track of my food intake or doing little or no exercise. But I don't keep thinking about the negative so much that it becomes ingrained in my mind and I automatically end up repeating it this week.

A few moments of quiet reflection with God clear my mind and prepare me to move on.

**"He reached down from on high, he took me;
he drew me out of mighty waters."
—Psalms 18:16**

Today's Message

Wonder of Life

My life is filled with wonder.

Life is a beautiful mystery. Gazing into the face of a child invokes a feeling of wonder within me. I see how precious life is.

Observing myself, I feel a sense of awe also. When I consider the intricacies of my own body and the complex functions it is capable of achieving, I am amazed. For instance, with a thought, my brain sends a message to my hand to pick something up: With seemingly little effort on my part, I watch as my arm reaches out and my fingers flex and curl around an object to move it. How wonderful my whole body is, and what wonder it performs!

The added wonder of my body is that it can adapt to change. So even after years of eating habits that have not been good for me, and no matter how much weight I may have put on, I still have the ability to make changes that will alter my appearance and improve my health. Yes, my life is filled with wonder!

"Call to me and I will answer you, and will tell you great and hidden things that you have not known."
—Jeremiah 33:3

Today's Message

Imagine That

Inspired by the wisdom of God, I expect to succeed and I do.

In my mind, I carry an image of what I will look like when I successfully reach my goal weight. When I am tempted to binge, I imagine that new me and thank God for the willpower to continue.

When I am in a situation in which it may be easy for me to overeat, I envision myself making healthy choices and eating only what I need.

On days when any exercise seems to be too much, I visualize myself moving more freely and having more energy. I imagine myself climbing stairs, riding a bicycle, or walking. Whatever I imagine, I am preparing myself to do. I thank God for the ability to both envision and accomplish something important to me.

My inspiration comes from God, and God knows and understands my every thought, dream, and hope. I can be successful in attaining what I have imagined because through the wisdom of God, I am being shown what I can do.

"The Lord searches every mind and understands every plan and thought."
—1 Chronicles 28:9

Today's Message

Smile

Each time I smile,
I bless my mind, body, and spirit.

I have made the amazing discovery that both of the following are equally true: smiling causes me to feel good and feeling good causes me to smile. No matter how difficult my day has been, when I turn a frown to a smile, I can't help but think happier thoughts. Even in the times when I feel discouraged, I have found that a smile uplifts me.

As I contemplate the expression: "Let a smile be your umbrella," I think about what it means. It's true: An open umbrella shields me from rain and keeps me dry and comfortable during a storm.

My smile acts like an umbrella, shielding me from negative feelings and thoughts. When I smile, I am coaching myself to think positive thoughts and have productive ideas. Each smile fills my heart with a warm, comfortable feeling that lifts my spirits and gives me courage to face any seeming obstacle.

"Happy are the people who know the festal shout,
who walk, O Lord, in the light of your countenance."
—Psalms 89:15

TODAY'S MESSAGE
Let Go, Let God

I let go and let God bring about perfect results.

I may have been advised to let go and let God when facing a challenge, but until now I didn't know what a powerful practice this is. I may have thought that letting go was giving up, but now I know that I am simply getting my own limited thoughts out of the way so that God can fill my mind with divine ideas.

I am no longer letting my actions get in the way of my own success; I am cooperating with God in bringing about perfect results.

When someone or some situation seems to be getting me down, I bless the person and the situation and turn everything over to God, saying: "Dear God, I don't know the answer to this challenge, but You do. So I am going to give it to You for a divine solution, knowing that You will let me know what You can do through me and others to heal the situation."

How calm I feel, letting go and letting God.

"But as for me, I will look to the Lord. I will wait for the God of my salvation; my God will hear me."
—Micah 7:7

MEDITATION

Listening

As God gently speaks to me,
I listen in reverence to a divine message.

Just as I make time in my day for exercise and relaxation, I also make time for meditation and prayer. At whatever time, day or night, I choose to meditate, I know that God is ready to listen.

I find a quiet place where I can easily calm myself and still my thoughts. As I close my eyes, I visualize every negative thought that I have brought with me taking flight. With my mind clear, I am aware that God is speaking to me.

I listen as God assures me of the divine love that is constantly being given to me. I don't even have to ask the questions on my heart. God gently answers them, and I listen in reverence to the divine wisdom I am receiving.

I allow God to be God in my life by listening to and then acting upon the guidance I receive.

"If then your whole body is full of light . . .
it will be as full of light as when a lamp
gives you light with its rays."
—Luke 11:36

◆ *Journal* ◆

Date: ______________________________

My weight: ______________________________

With God, my family,
and my friends supporting me,
I am a winner.

I am also a winner because ______________

____

____

____

____

____

____

____

____

____

____

Today's Message

Courage

Prayer is a powerful way that I receive the courage to do my best.

I needed courage to step onto the scale and weigh myself when I first started my weight-loss program or when I strayed from following it. Yet when I was with a group of friends or others, who, like me, were trying to lose weight, I felt encouraged. In fact, just being with one another and talking about what helped us encouraged us all.

Being with people who are working toward the same or similar goals, I feel more courageous. Perhaps there is courage in numbers. Maybe it's because we know the importance of what we are doing, and we silently and verbally support each other in doing our best.

I believe there is a mighty power released when two or more pray together and for one another. Whenever I am able to say "no" to a huge piece of my favorite dessert, just maybe someone is praying for me at that very moment, reinforcing my courage.

"Each one helps the other,
saying to one another, 'Take courage!'"
—Isaiah 41:6

TODAY'S MESSAGE

Child of God

—◆—

I am a child of God who is loved unconditionally and sustained eternally by God.

As a child of God, I honor the sacred responsibility of taking good care of myself. By listening to my Creator, I know what I need to do and how to go about doing it. God is my loving, eternal parent who guides me every moment of every day. And as God's child, I listen to and follow the divine wisdom I receive.

Divine guidance helps me know which dieting approach works for me. If I have a craving for sweets, I remember that there are fresh fruits such as apples, grapes, or oranges that will satisfy my craving and fill that empty spot in my stomach.

God and I share a sacred bond that can never be broken and a divine communication that no other person can hear. I rejoice in the understanding of who I am: a child of God who is loved unconditionally and sustained eternally.

"As he who called you is holy, be holy yourselves in all your conduct; for it is written, 'You shall be holy, for I am holy.'"
—1 Peter 1:15–16

TODAY'S MESSAGE

Hope

—◆—

Because of God, I always have hope.

Hope is a sacred attitude of heart and soul. Such an attitude proclaims that good is possible and encourages me to live my life believing that the possibility will become a reality.

Hope tells me that I can add a couple of blocks to my daily walk, be a few or several pounds lighter soon, and once again fit into my favorite outfit.

Hope encourages me to have patience with myself and to stay inspired so that I continue to make progress.

I know what hope is and does for me. And what gives me hope is that continuing echo of something God whispered to me: "You can do this, for I am with you, loving you and supporting you in every moment." I have hope, because of God. Or maybe it's better said: Because of God, I always have hope.

"For in hope we were saved. Now hope that is seen
is not hope. For who hopes for what is seen?
But if we hope for what we do not see,
we wait for it with patience."
—Romans 8:24

Today's Message

Serenity

—◆—

God within enables me to be serene and to live a life of peace.

God, who is at the center of the universe, is also at the center of my being. Because I am attuned to the peace of God within me, I release that peace and let it flow throughout my being.

The feeling of serenity I experience when I cooperate with God is a peace that is unshakable. God is the divine wisdom that guides me as I make decisions concerning the food I eat and the physical activities that I undertake.

God is the still, small voice that proclaims a message of hope and reassurance. I go to God within to be in touch with divine intelligence and understanding, for God is the source of all that I need to live a life of peace.

I am always in a state of transition, making a vital move forward in knowing greater and greater peace. With God as my constant guide and companion, I am a serene and secure being.

"Know that I am with you."
—Genesis 28:15

Today's Message

Rejuvenated

Prayer rejuvenates my mind and strengthens my resolve.

After a day of following my diet and taking the time to exercise properly, I feel good about myself and what I have accomplished. That rejuvenating feeling is one that I want to keep up each day.

So if I feel tempted to snack while watching television or to head for the refrigerator after an upsetting situation, I remember how good I felt when I had accomplished my daily goals.

Then I turn to God for strength rather than turning to the refrigerator. I use prayer rather than food as an energizer, and I feel rejuvenated. Whenever I still feel hungry after eating a meal, I pray for 10 to 15 minutes and focus my attention on God. After the time has passed, the hunger probably will be gone. If it hasn't, I now have the inner strength to make a wise choice rather than grabbing the first thing that looks good to me. Again, I know the feeling of accomplishment!

"The God of all grace . . . will himself restore, support, strengthen, and establish you."
—1 Peter 5:10

TODAY'S MESSAGE
Healthy and Whole

—◆—

I am transforming my lifestyle to a healthier and more complete way of living.

When I made the decision to live healthier, I took a step forward in transforming my lifestyle to one that is healthy and whole. Eating right and maintaining a level of physical activity is a lifetime commitment, one that I do not take lightly.

I appreciate life and want to do whatever helps me in living a healthier, more complete life. I look to God for guidance in realizing any changes that I may need to make in my attitude and for the encouragement that inspires me to move toward the realization of my hopes and dreams.

To be sure that I am cooperating, I become an observer of myself. I may keep a diary, writing down and keeping track of everything I eat throughout the day. I may find an exercise buddy—a friend to talk to as we workout or walk together.

The changes I make now will affect my life in positive ways today and in the future.

"Prepare your work outside, get everything ready for you in the field; and after that build your house."
—Proverbs 24:27

MEDITATION

Healing

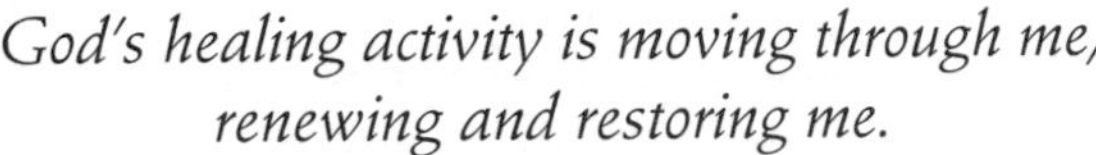

God's healing activity is moving through me, renewing and restoring me.

Although my meditation today may be time of physical *inactivity* for me, it is a time of sacred *activity* for my soul. In this time of rest for my body, I call forth a healing energy that springs from the spirit of God at the center of my being.

Quieting my body and every thought but ones of health, I gently affirm: *God's healing activity is moving through me, renewing and restoring me*. I affirm that my metabolism and immune system are working in perfect order and that my heart is sending nourishment throughout my body.

Attuned to the healing activity that is within me, I want to cooperate with it now and at all other times. So as I go back to the activity of my day, I continue to affirm life and healing, and I thank God that the sacred activity of my soul is ongoing.

"My child, be attentive to my words; incline your ear to my sayings . . . For they are life to those who find them, and healing to all their flesh."
—Proverbs 4:20

◆ *Journal* ◆

Date: ______________________________

My weight: ___________________________

I am aware that I am making progress in matters large and small.

Things that I can do to reward myself may include buying a new outfit, taking time to read a good book, or ______________________

____

____

____

____

____

____

____

____

____

Today's Message

Fresh Look

I take a fresh look at myself and see the possibilities.

I am in awe of God's creative, sustaining power, and when I take a fresh look at myself through faith-filled eyes, I know that God has created me with the potential for wonderful possibilities. Keeping that potential in mind, I don't become discouraged.

Because I know that one possibility is for me to lose unwanted pounds, which in turn will improve my appearance and my health, I envision myself as I will look after I have reduced to a smaller size. I am taking a fresh look at myself. Thinking of the person I would like to be helps bolster my self-esteem and my resolve to succeed.

I visualize myself as graceful and strong. With this picture in my mind and knowing that with God's help it is attainable, I remain focused on doing and eating what is healthy and good for me.

"For now we see in a mirror, dimly, but then we will see face to face. Now I know only in part; then I will know fully, even as I have been fully known."
—1 Corinthians 13:12

Today's Message
Responsible

I am a responsible person—
toward others and toward myself.

When did I feel most responsible? Was it when my parents handed me the car keys for my first solo drive? Or was it that magical moment when I first held my newborn baby in my arms? Those times I felt both awe and apprehension. I wanted to take on both roles but knew they required great responsibility. Maybe realizing this made me a better driver and parent.

Throughout life, I want to honor my responsibilities toward others. Yet I am also committed to myself. When I accept some responsibility for my own health and well-being, I think and do things that benefit me in the way I look, feel, and move about. For instance, my food choices are based on what maintains and enhances my health. My activities are ones that strengthen my heart and fulfill me.

In being a responsible person, I am willing to bless others and I am also willing to bless myself.

"Restore to me the joy of your salvation,
and sustain in me a willing spirit."
—Psalms 51:12

Today's Message

Satisfied Soul

God alone satisfies my soul.

Some days my progress may not show on the scale or in the way my clothes fit or in my energy level. The most important improvement that can happen may be more intangible, and that is what is happening within my head and my heart—even deep within my soul.

This kind of change for the better comes from God. With God as my companion and guide, I am able to rise above habits from the past and replace them with more healthful ways of thinking, eating, and living. Then I know how rewarding it is not to feel desperate at the sight or smell of a potato chip or rich dessert!

So how do I measure my progress? The satisfaction deep within my soul is the true measure of my spiritual and emotional growth. With each step I take, I feel God's loving presence guiding me along my chosen path—a pathway to wholeness—and I am filled with thanksgiving.

"My soul is satisfied as with a rich feast, and my mouth praises you with joyful lips."
—Psalms 63:5

Today's Message

Zest for Living

My spirit is light and my heart is free, for I have a new zest for living.

I have found a new zest for living!

Over the past weeks, I have made strides toward attaining my ideal weight. I have practiced a new and wholesome lifestyle by eating a variety of healthy foods and exercising regularly. And with each pound I shed, I have gained a greater zest for living.

Yes, my body weight is becoming lighter, but so is my spirit. I feel freer than ever before. I am light-hearted, happy, and enthusiastic about life.

My zest for living is an expression of the spirit of God within me. This same spirit guides and strengthens me and helps me as I aspire to reach my goal and express myself in new, enriching ways.

With my new-found zest for living, I look forward to new adventures. I know that I can do whatever I want or need to do, so I step out with courage and faith to participate fully in life.

**"I will be glad and exult in you;
I will sing praise to your name, O Most High."
—Psalms 9:2**

Today's Message

Positive Investment

Using my time and resources wisely, I make a positive investment in my well-being.

My time and my resources are precious gifts from God. So what will I invest them in today? When I invest my time in physical activities that strengthen my body, I am taking steps to improve my well-being.

The same is true when I invest my thoughts in making wise choices about food. I am using wisdom in a way that satisfies the cells and tissues of my body and keeps them strong and whole.

My good health benefits not only me, it also benefits the people who depend on me. The more energy and vitality I have, the more I can be there for my family, friends, and coworkers.

I invest my time and thoughts in God. These sacred moments fill me with infinite calm, which comes from a limitless reservoir of peace within me. I allow the tranquility I feel to radiate from me and to harmonize my relationships with others.

"Let your gifts be for yourself."
—Daniel 5:17

TODAY'S MESSAGE

Today

I understand how blessed I am to be me!

Today I acknowledge the progress I am making. I take my focus off weight and food and concentrate on enjoying today.

I reward myself by scheduling time to do what I want to do—whether it is going on a shopping trip or starting a craft project. I have earned a day for myself and I would be remiss in passing up an opportunity to indulge in healthy, satisfying activities.

Today I can take a brisk walk and feel a oneness with God's creation. Listening to birds sing or the laughter of children, I hear in each note a chord that calls on me to respond with feelings of joy. I thank God for a beautiful day that is filled with sights and sounds of creation.

Today I acknowledge what I have accomplished and who I am. I am worthy of this day, and I step forth in faith to enjoy it. I understand how blessed I am to be me!

"The time is fulfilled, and the kingdom of God has come near . . . believe in the good news."
—Mark 1:15

MEDITATION

Blessed Assurance

The assurance of God's presence satisfies me—spirit, mind, and body.

I take a few moments now to be alone with God. I find a place where I will not be disturbed. I may choose to sit in a comfortable chair, but wherever I choose to be in this sacred time, I begin to relax. I shrug my shoulders and flex my ankles. Then I allow my body to completely relax.

I imagine that I am moving into a place of light and beauty, of peace and quiet. I listen for and hear the invitation: "Welcome, beloved. I am here with you now and I assure you that I am with you always."

The assurance of God's presence revives me; I breathe deeply and relax even more. I realize that what I might have thought of as a hunger for food was a desire to be totally in the presence of God. Assured of God's presence, I feel a satisfaction of my total being—spirit, body, and soul.

"Now faith is the assurance of things hoped for, the conviction of things not seen."
—Hebrews 11:1

♦ *Journal* ♦

Date: ________________________________

My weight: ____________________________

I explore new ways
I can bring a greater variety
to my weight-loss program.

I try a new low-fat recipe, exchange helpful ideas on weight loss with a friend, or ________

____

____

____

____

____

____

____

____

____

Today's Message

Wake Up!

—◆—

I am awake to the variety of life.

Sometimes I may seem to be on automatic pilot because my life is routine. Then in a moment of realization, I understand that God is giving me a wake-up call to life. I feel an inner urging to step outside my usual comfort zone and know that life is never routine. Changes are happening everywhere.

Awakened to life, I welcome color and texture and newness into my day. Simple changes can affect me in dramatic ways. For instance, I realize that my food tastes better when I eat a meal off my "special" china. By adding the colors and textures of a variety of vegetables to a salad, I enhance the flavor of the salad and my satisfaction in eating it.

God has created a world of wonder and guides me in experiencing the variety of life every day. I never become bored, because I know that life is offering me an ever-changing panorama of choices.

"Our friend Lazarus has fallen asleep, but I am going there to wake him."
—John 11:11

TODAY'S MESSAGE

Potential

My real potential is to be healthy and to be happy with who I am.

There is the potential of a tall oak tree within one small round acorn, and there is the potential of a slimmer me within my present shape and form. There is much more I want to achieve than looks, however—although I will accept that kind of improvement. Most important, I can improve my health and the way I feel.

That potential of weighing less is possible, because I am not relying totally on my own willpower; I am relying on God-power. The power of God can shape my potential into reality, and I call on God for strength and wisdom to do what I need to achieve success.

Losing weight will help my heart, my joints, and my flexibility. I also know that my ideal weight will differ from that of others. I am relying on God to help me bring out my best, and I thank God that my true potential is taking shape day by day.

"For mortals it is impossible, but for God all things are possible."
—Matthew 19:26

Today's Message

Indomitable Spirit

Just by continuing to try, I am succeeding.

Even though I feel as if I am taking two steps back for each step forward in trying to achieve something, I remain optimistic. I know in my heart that the only true failure is in not trying at all.

So if I have not stayed with my diet today, rather than tear myself down, I affirm that I will try again tomorrow. God has blessed me with an indomitable spirit, and I know that I can and will succeed.

The spirit of God within me will help me rise above any physical challenge with a resurgence of spiritual strength. Together, God and I are masters of my life.

Although I want to lose a certain amount of weight, I know that it will not happen overnight. Through my indomitable spirit I am investing time in the care and keeping of my body. Step by step, I am continually succeeding because I am continuing to try.

"But as for that in the good soil, these are the ones who, when they hear the word, hold it fast in an honest and good heart, and bear fruit with patient endurance."
—Luke 8:15

Today's Message

Simple Words

—◆—

Words of love, faith, and hope inspire and encourage me in living a healthful, vigorous life.

There is power in words, and simple, familiar words speak to me in a powerful, uplifting way. Words such as *love*, *faith*, and *hope* build me up and prepare me to move beyond what I think I can do to accomplish even more.

I know this as I continue to improve my health. I have come a long way and even though I have a ways to go before I reach my target weight, I have faith that I will not only reach it, I will maintain it.

I eliminate thoughts and words that would limit me in any endeavor I am committed to. God loves me, and I love myself as God's creation. I have faith in God and faith in myself. I have hope for good results that inspires and encourages me onward.

My positive, life-affirming words support me in continuing on with and then in sustaining a healthful and vigorous life.

"The teacher sought to find pleasing words, and he wrote words of truth plainly."
—Ecclesiastes 12:10

Today's Message
Acceptance

—◆—

I accept myself as someone who has been lovingly and wonderfully created by God.

I am a unique creation, different from any other being on Earth. I may follow the same food plan as a friend and not lose as much weight as she does. My metabolism may be operating at a different rate. I accept that.

Although I follow my diet and exercise regularly, sometimes I do not see any measurable success. I may weigh the same as others and still not look as thin as they look. I accept that.

If I do not meet another's expectations, still I know that I am doing what is right for me. I accept that.

I accept my difference in appearance and the different ways my body reacts to dieting and exercise because I know that I have been lovingly and wonderfully created by God.

With this assurance, I continue to eat wisely and exercise to stay fit, knowing that one day, I will look in the mirror and say, "I accept that!"

"I praise you, for I am . . . wonderfully made."
—Psalms 139:14

TODAY'S MESSAGE

Celebration

—◆—

I am a work in progress, and with a grateful heart, I celebrate my accomplishments.

Some of the happiest times of my life have involved celebrations, for they marked important milestones.

Throughout the past few weeks, I have achieved milestones as I undertook a weight-loss program. I have learned new habits, found new strengths, and formed new attitudes.

These milestones deserve a celebration, a special recognition. I may wish to celebrate them by watching a favorite movie, taking a relaxing stroll, reading a cherished book, or spending time with a friend. My celebrations are personal rewards for a job well done, a job that I continue each day.

I celebrate my accomplishments and the blessings of my experiences. There are new tasks and new opportunities to celebrate before me. I look forward to these experiences with confidence and with the anticipation of celebrating them with family and friends.

"With gratitude in your hearts sing psalms, hymns, and spiritual songs to God."
—Colossians 3:16

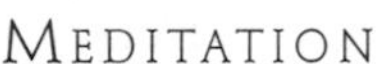

MEDITATION

Motivation

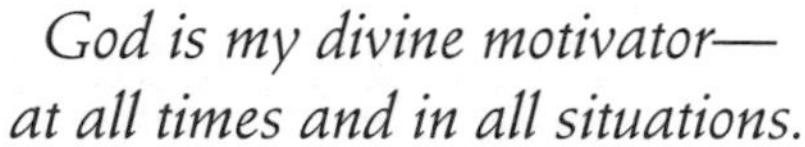

*God is my divine motivator—
at all times and in all situations.*

Only a moment or two of meditation time motivates me. For instance, when I am in a social situation where foods on my diet plan are not available, I turn to God for motivation to keep from over-indulging. While looking at a menu or waiting in line for a buffet—with eyes wide open—I silently turn within to God:

"Dear God, thank You for this opportunity to share a meal with good friends. I am open right now to Your guidance in selecting a meal that is healthy and as close as possible to my eating program. You motivate me to eat right portions. Thank You, God, for encouraging me."

As I move forward in line or choose my meal from the menu, I end my time of quiet meditation and feel a great peace about my selections.

**"We walk by faith, not by sight."
—2 Corinthians 5:7**

◆ *Journal* ◆

Date: ______________________________

My weight: ______________________________

I explore new avenues
for varying my exercise routine.

I can park farther from the store so that I have farther to walk, or I can ____________________

____

____

____

____

____

____

____

____

____

____

Use this relaxation technique to stay calm or relaxed. It is simple to do and can be done just about anywhere:

Sit or lay down in a comfortable position. Keeping your mouth closed, inhale slowly through your nose. (Your stomach area should rise as you inhale.)

Exhale slowly through your mouth. (Your stomach should go down as you exhale.) Repeat three or four times or until you feel calm or relaxed.

◆

SOURCE: *Shape Up America! Support Center*

The Faith to Overcome

By Colleen Zuck

Growing up, I often heard my mother remark: "We may be poor, but we never go hungry." There was always plenty of food and plenty of love in my family's home. Yet hunger had been a real issue in my mother's family when she was a child: Her father had deserted his family, leaving my grandmother with eight children to raise on her own. The oldest child was about 16; the youngest, 6 months old.

My mother and her brothers and sisters went to work as soon as they were old enough to earn money. One of my uncles started work in a lime mine when he was just 7 years old. I remember hearing stories of how they subsisted on water gravy—a bit of lard and flour thinned with water—for sometimes a week at a time. Making a living in the hills of northwestern Arkansas in the 1920s was difficult indeed. For a woman with little education and eight children, it was a matter of survival—every day.

Yes, hunger had been a huge problem for my mother's family, and somehow I came to believe that by avoiding hunger, I could avoid problems. I developed an added twist to this theory: Whenever I had a problem, the more I ate, the less the problem or life itself could hurt me. Just before the new millennium, I was literally carrying around over 60 pounds of extra weight.

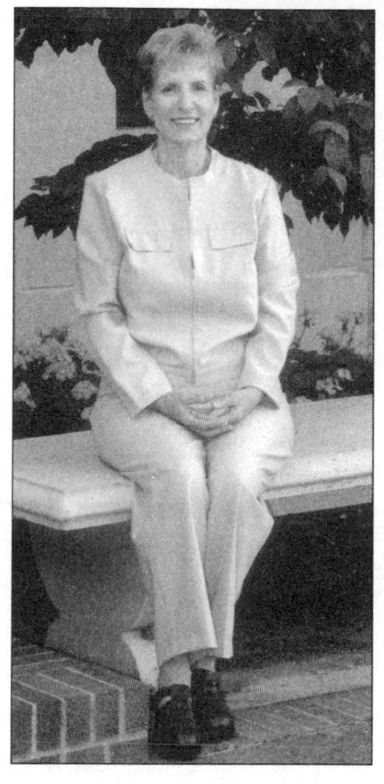

Oh, I had lost weight several times over my lifetime, but gained even more weight back each time. I was an avid picture taker, but if at all possible, I never allowed my picture to be taken. I didn't like the way I looked, and of even more importance, I didn't feel well. The pain in my hip joints increased with my weight gain. I prayed about losing weight, but I was expecting God to do for me what I was perfectly capable of doing myself.

Problems didn't go away, no matter how much I ate. My father was diagnosed with Alzheimer's disease. Over the next 3 years, Mom took care of Dad, and other family members and I helped Mom. My grown son John had an apartment in my parents' house and was faithful in watching over his grandparents.

During the final 3 months of his life, Dad needed constant care—day and night. So he spent that time in a nursing home. We visited him daily, but his absence in the home created a cloud of gloom over our family.

A couple of years after Dad passed, Mom was also diagnosed with Alzheimer's. She was living alone by then, and her short-term memory was drastically affected. I noticed that her beautiful collie had gained a lot of weight. On my visits to her each day, I counted the empty dog food cans—up to six in one single day! Then I knew: Forgetting that she had fed him, she fed him repeatedly throughout the day.

Although Mom's memory was slipping away, her sense of humor and appetite grew stronger. She, too, gained weight. As I began helping her with her checkbook, I discovered that she was ordering a pizza five times a week. Other problems came to light, and my brothers and I decided her health and safety were in jeopardy if she continued living alone.

I expected Mom to agree to move in with me. We had not only been close as mother and daughter, we had also been the best of friends. However, the more I insisted on a move, the more Mom resisted. I think she was aware that her condition was even worse than what we knew it to be. Finally my brothers and I agreed that we had to move her out of her home. She would stay with my husband, Bill, and me, Friday through Sunday (when I was off work) and with my brother Richard and his wife, Pauline, Monday through Thursday.

We did this for about 2 years, but Mom's confusion produced frightening consequences: She wandered around the house at night and, despite locks and gates, she got out of the house during the day. On one such occasion, she was missing from my brother's house, and he found her walking up the street. After that we decided that Mom needed more care than any of us or all of us together could give her.

The next step—placing her in a long-term Alzheimer's facility—was one of the hardest decisions I had ever had to make, and I know my brothers felt the same. I anguished over this move and continued to overeat. Somehow I was using food as my comfort—so that I would feel better. The opposite was true; the more weight I gained, the worse I felt.

Mother's extra weight made it harder for her walk. Eventually it became so difficult for her to walk that she didn't. With little or no physical activity, she gained more weight even though she was eating less food.

I was about at the end of my rope one day when my son, John, telephoned. "Mom, I am enrolling in Weight Watcher's class. Do you want to join, too?" When I answered *yes* to that invitation, I took control of my life. Over the next year, John lost over 90 pounds, and I lost over 60!

Of course the food plan, motivational topics, and camaraderie of the group helped me. But a simple, practical statement the instructor made really held a picture of myself in front of my eyes. She offered this question to the class: "When you feel stress building over a problem, do you really believe that eating a bag of potato chips or half a dozen cookies will solve the problem?" Every head in the room shook "no." We knew it would only add to our problems.

This example offered some practical insight that was supported by spiritual insight. I prayed to have the faith to overcome and make it through problems—from aggravation to crisis. Problems happen in life, and how I dealt with them made the difference. I realized that I was responsible for how I ate and what I ate, if I exercised and how often I exercised.

Three months after I had reached my weight-loss goal, my faith and my willingness to be responsible were tested. John was scheduled for surgery. A biopsy would be done, but the doctor believed the growth on John's larynx was benign. I felt an immediate bond with the kind nurse who was preparing John for surgery. As we talked, I learned that like me, she read *Daily Word* magazine every day. Within an hour, I was to learn something else: Nancy was there by divine appointment.

I was so stunned, I could hardly think or talk when the doctor told us the growth was malignant. Nancy stood in the corner taking notes. She seemed to read my mind and my heart, making arrangements for me to stay with John at the hospital that night. The next morning, she came to visit John and rejoiced with us over the good news about tests done the night before: The cancer had not spread.

John was presented with two options: He could have his voice box removed and radiation, or he could have radiation twice a day for 6 weeks with 3 weeks of chemotherapy. John chose treatment rather than surgery.

I knew with greater clarity than ever before that it would be love and prayer and faith that would bring us all through this time. And this is what happened. All tests show that John is healed. I have been so blessed witnessing the healing power of God work wonders through John.

And through it all, I didn't slip back into an old pattern of overeating. What I had learned and practiced about eating healthy, nutritious foods in right proportions was so much a part of my daily routine that I continued to make wise choices.

On my one-year anniversary of meeting my weight-loss goal, John called to congratulate me: "Mom, I am so proud of you for losing weight and for keeping it off." That was a great compliment coming from someone I loved so dearly.

The greatest gift of all was that I had heard my son speaking in a voice that was clear and strong. Thank God; how truly satisfied I felt.

Today's Message

Feeling of Satisfaction

God is my unfailing help and strength, my unending source of satisfaction and fulfillment.

In the past, I may have tried to find some kind of appeasement and gratification through the food I ate, but by doing this, I never truly felt satisfied or complete. Over the past few months, however, I have found new ways in which to feel the satisfaction, the sense of wholeness I have been looking for.

I have a newly discovered soul-satisfaction that comes from turning my dreams and desires over to God and opening myself to God's fulfilling love. God is my unfailing help and strength, my unending source of satisfaction and fulfillment.

I have gained a new sense of peace and a deeper understanding of myself as a spiritual being with physical needs. Yet even those needs are fulfilled as I turn to God, the true source of all fulfillment.

I have experienced a wonderful contentment. This feeling fills my soul and flows throughout my being and every area of my life.

"And my God will fully satisfy every need of yours."
—Philippians 4:18

Today's Message

Youthful Spirit

I am young and vitally alive through the life-giving spirit of God within me and around me.

When I watch younger people interact with each other, I may say, "If only I had their energy!" While being young is a chronological fact, it is an attitudinal one as well.

I can always choose to have youthful spirit—one that inspires me to have energy and vitality. How? By realizing that I am filled with the life-giving spirit of God. The spirit of God has created me, and the presence of God's spirit fills me with strength and vitality.

Right now, I take a deep breath and breathe in the breath of life, for the spirit of God that is present within me is also in the very air that surrounds me. As I breathe in, I experience a surge of energy. I do feel younger and vitally alive.

Ready to face the day with joy in my heart, I can hardly contain the youthful sense of wonder and excitement for what is about to unfold today.

"The spirit of God has made me,
and the breath of the Almighty gives me life."
—Job 33:4

Today's Message

Where I Am

Wherever I am, whatever I do, God is my guide, my strength, and my companion.

I have adopted new ways of thinking, eating, and exercising, learning along the way what brings about the greatest results. I continue to make progress by continuing in these ways and by looking for new ways to maintain my positive self-image.

If ever I feel my resolve slipping, however, I review some of the things that helped me get to this point. As I renew my commitment to God and myself, I also renew my determination to stay with the plan that has worked so well for me.

I am happy with myself and my success, yet I know that the changes I continue to make contribute to a happier, healthier life for me. I am eager to explore new expressions that reflect a positive attitude.

I thank God for helping me get where I am, and for the wisdom and inspiration to know what is best for me in each new tomorrow.

"Continue in what you have learned and firmly believed, knowing from whom you learned it."
—2 Timothy 3:14

TODAY'S MESSAGE

In Tune

***In tune with God's love,
I express a symphony of praise to God.***

The music of a symphony orchestra is an intricately woven tapestry of melody, rhythm, and harmony. To produce the finest tone quality, orchestra members tune their instruments carefully so that the music they play delights the ear.

I want the quality of my life to be like a symphony orchestra. At the beginning of each day, I make sure that I am in tune by attuning myself to the perfection of God's love that keeps me happy, wise, and whole.

In quiet moments, I feel the love of God stirring within me, playing on the heartstrings of my soul. I am confident that divine love will harmonize and direct my thoughts and actions, helping me keep my mind clear and my body fit. I am in tune with God's love.

The soothing symphony playing within me is a song of praise to God, and it fills me with peace.

"Praise the Lord with the lyre; make melody to him with the harp of ten strings. Sing to him a new song; play skillfully on the strings, with loud shouts."
—Psalms 33:2–3

Today's Message

In This Moment

—◆—

In this moment, I explore the depths of my soul and the abundance of my blessings.

In this moment . . .

I accept that I have yet untapped reservoirs of strength and ability. I see myself as an achiever and do not question what heights of achievement I can reach.

I live from the assurance of God's presence, which resides within me as life and intelligence, as spirit and power. I am courageous and confident.

I know without a doubt that now is the time to release all resentment and anger. I don't mistreat myself or accept it from others as something I deserve. I deserve to be loved and valued.

I embrace all this moment holds for me by thinking positive thoughts and feeling serene. This is a time of giving thanks for my blessings and for opening my mind and my life to even greater ones.

Now is the time for me to live life fully—one moment, one day at a time.

"See, now is the acceptable time;
see, now is the day of salvation."
—2 Corinthians 6:2

TODAY'S MESSAGE

Keeping It Simple

God is my support, a constant presence of wisdom and power that blesses me.

Life can be complicated enough at times, so I do not add to it with something as unproductive as worrying. I keep my life simple and uncomplicated by relying on the wisdom and strength of God to fulfill me.

God is the compass that guides me. God understands that I may hesitate at times, uncertain as to what I should do. But I hear God's gentle words of assurance resounding within me and feel my Creator's presence nudging me in the way that I should go.

I lean on God when I need support. In God's presence I find the reassurance I seek. While every moment may not be as effortless to live through as I would hope, I relax, knowing that God is with me.

I am thankful that I can choose to turn every concern over to God for the right and perfect solution.

**"Worship the Lord with gladness;
come into his presence with singing."
—Psalms 100:2**

Meditation
Sacred Retreat

I journey within on a sacred retreat where I am one with God.

A retreat is a place I can go to escape the "busyness" of life. As I turn within for a sacred retreat, I turn away from the hustle and bustle around me and turn to the powerful presence of God.

I settle in a comfortable chair, close my eyes, and still my thoughts. As I focus on the holy Presence within, I no longer hear the sounds around me. In a blessed surrender, I open the way for God to fill my entire being. I drift further away from the physical world and into the spiritual realm.

In the silence, I find inner beauty and a purpose for being. All tension leaves my body, and I rest. I feel a lightness of being, a sensation of being held gently and lovingly. Here in this sacred retreat, I am in touch with the eternal oneness of God, and I know how truly blessed I am.

"I will instruct you and teach you."
—Psalms 32:8

• *Journal* •

Date: __________________________________

My weight: ______________________________

I know that burning calories
helps keep me energized and healthy.

I can burn more calories by walking, jogging, or

Today's Message

Now Is the Time

—◆—

Now is the time for my soul to rejoice!

Now is the time to enjoy every moment of life. What better time than now to recognize and give thanks for the beauty and power of God that shine forth from me as love and compassion.

Now is the time for me to let my friends and loved ones know just how much they mean to me and the many ways they have blessed me. Now is a golden opportunity to let others know of my love for them.

Now is the time to give thanks for what was, what is, and whatever will be. I am a link in the circle of life that spans the globe, and I feel a divine connection with all creation.

Now is the time for me to expand my mind by being open to the unlimited possibilities that await me.

Now is a time for my soul to rejoice for the wondrous blessings that God has given me.

"I will sing praises to my God all my life long."
—Psalms 146:2

Today's Message

New Self-Image

—◆—

I am a healthy, happy child of God.

Who is this new me that I wake up to each morning and walk with each day? Who is this person with more energy, different eating habits, new desires for activity?

Each day, I thank God for the new person I am becoming physically, emotionally, and spiritually. I take delight in a new feeling of freedom, a new level of energy, a new sense of fashion, and a renewed faith in God to direct me.

As I become more accustomed to looking and feeling differently, I am aware that it is God's uncompromising love that upholds me. I thank God for creating within me the desire to turn away from unhealthy habits and embrace new ones.

I trust God to guide me in being wise, loving, and patient as I accept my new self-image and make it a part of my everyday life.

"You have stripped off the old self with its practices and have clothed yourselves with the new self, which is being renewed in knowledge according to the image of its creator."
—Colossians 3:9–10

Today's Message

Special Day

I appreciate this day, and my appreciation makes it a special day.

How long has it been since I have given myself the gift of a special day? I think it is time I did—today!

What do I most want to do? Maybe I will take extra time to meditate on the presence of God and recharge my spiritual battery. Recharged spiritually, I can take on my day with enthusiasm for whatever I do.

After some quiet reflection, I may want to burn some calories. A brisk walk or bike ride through my neighborhood would invigorate me and give me a chance to wave and say *hi* to some of my neighbors.

Spending time with loved ones can be just what I need to make this day special. An impromptu call to someone, extending an invitation to visit the zoo or see a play could make this a special day for both of us. Regardless of what I do today, I want to show my appreciation to God for the very day itself. Every day becomes special when I am thankful for it.

"I am about to do a new thing; now it springs forth, do you not perceive it?"
—Isaiah 43:19

Today's Message

Healthy Lifestyle

—◆—

My positive thoughts and cheerful disposition keep me on the path of good health.

My cheerful disposition keeps me from taking myself too seriously and brightens my outlook on life. My positive thoughts lead to constructive actions that are sweet indeed, for they remind me that I am divinely designed to be healthy, happy, and strong.

I want to continue enjoying the benefits of being fit physically, so I nourish my body with nutritious food and plenty of water and exercise.

I know that staying mentally fit means that I nourish my mind, learning something new every day. Reading and writing, listening and watching, and other activities keep my mind alert and active.

The most positive thing I can do in nourishing my soul is to set aside time each day for quiet times of prayer and meditation. These moments draw me closer in awareness to God and promote my overall health and well-being.

"Pleasant words are like a honeycomb, sweetness to the soul and health to the body."
—Proverbs 16:24

Today's Message

Flexible

I thank God that I am flexible.

So much of life is about adapting when the unexpected happens. Being flexible, I have learned that I can adapt when my plans or expectations take a different turn. This flexibility has been a great help to me in losing weight and in maintaining my weight loss.

I have learned so much about making wise food choices and how adapting recipes to include low-fat, low-sugar ingredients will still produce a tasty, satisfying meal. I have learned that being less rigid in my expectations of myself has given me more peace of mind. I then am able to continue coaching myself in making healthy, wise choices.

I can because God is continually giving me the understanding and the strength to make the best of what may seem the worst of circumstances. Flexibility enables me to succeed and to enjoy what I am doing to make that possible.

"Whoever becomes humble like this child is the greatest in the kingdom of heaven."
—Matthew 18:4

Today's Message

Amazing Me

I am an example of God's creativity, and I live my life as the amazing creation that I am.

How would I feel if someone were to say that I am an amazing person? Let me say this about myself and experience my own feelings: "I am amazing!" Do I feel a bit embarrassed? Am I saying something that is true about me?

The answer to the first question may be *yes*; however, the answer to the second question is absolutely *yes*! It's true; I am amazing. My greatness is in being a child of God and living from my true identity.

God's creative power is amazing and so is everyone and everything that God has created. When I accept that this is true about me, I won't hold myself back from accomplishing goals and from keeping true to them for years to come.

I am amazing, because God has created me. Knowing this, I live my life as the amazing creation of God that I am.

"So God created humankind in his image, in the image of God he created them."
—Genesis 1:27

MEDITATION

Spiritual Foundation

I am secure, for I am building my life on a solid foundation of faith and prayer.

Gently, I close my eyes and relax my body. I project an image of myself as I am now on the screen of my mind. Am I satisfied with how I look?

Maybe I want to lose just a few more pounds. Now I ask myself how I get from here to there.

Maybe I am at that perfect weight, so my self-picture is of me now. Do I feel secure about remaining at this weight? Or do I worry that I can't?

I now take in the bigger picture and see that I have the foundation of my faith in God supporting me. Each time I have acted in faith, each time I have prayed has made my foundation for a full and satisfying life even stronger.

My spiritual foundation is solid, and I am sure that I can lose more or remain the same weight. In a few minutes, I have refreshed my confidence and faith.

"Come, you that are blessed by my Father, inherit the kingdom prepared for you from the foundation of the world."
—Matthew 25:34

◆ *Journal* ◆

Date: ______________________________

My weight: __________________________

Eating more than I need may give me temporary pleasure, but it can result in unwanted pounds and inches later.

My true sources of comfort are my family, friends, and __________________________

____

____

____

____

____

____

____

____

____

TODAY'S MESSAGE

Wellness

—◆—

***Filled with an awareness of God,
I realize that I am well and strong.***

In the past few weeks, I have become more aware of myself, my spirituality, and what it means to be whole and well. I have come to realize that being well is more than a physical experience; it is also a spiritual one.

I know that to be well is to be healthy and strong in mind and body, but it is much more than that. It is also the sense of security I have in who I am and where I am going with my life. I feel this sense of security, embracing each day as a new opportunity to experience God on a deeper level—a level of true wholeness in spirit, mind, and body.

Through my growing awareness of God, I am building trust in myself to act wisely in regard to my health and well-being. As I give myself, heart and soul, to God, I realize that I am whole and well in every way. I also know how to support that wholeness by what I think, say, and do.

**"Teach me the way I should go,
for to you I lift up my soul."
—Psalms 143:8**

Today's Message

Strength of Spirit

—◆—

I have a strength of spirit that builds my confidence in making further progress.

If at any time I feel that, for some unexplainable reason, I have stalled and cannot move forward with my plan for healthy living, I know that God will support me so that I can continue on. My faith assures me that the way out of a challenging situation is to see my way through it and that God will be with me all the way.

Having met and overcome the challenge, I discover that I am stronger and that my faith is renewed. All this is the result of a strength of spirit that builds confidence. I am able to face this day and every day with assurance.

Despite what is taking place around me, I am serene at the core of my innermost being, and my spirit is strong. I give thanks that God is in charge in my life and in my world and that God's presence strengthens me each day. I have the strength of spirit to move on.

"Do you not know that you are God's temple and that God's Spirit dwells in you?"
—1 Corinthians 3:16

Today's Message

Worthy

God assures me that I am worthy, for I am a divine creation.

When I put myself and my worth in true perspective, I understand that I am worthy of every blessing, every good, every success that could be. God deemed me worthy of being created, or I would not be here on Earth. So if God regards me as someone of great value, how can I not value myself!

There are heights and depths to me that I have yet to discover and explore. Because I value myself, I want to do what is best for me concerning my health and the very quality of my life.

I can and do bring quality to my life and enhance my health by the way I think and act. Nourishing food and physical activity are probably the nearest things to the mythical fountain of youth. I am worthy of being healthy and vigorous. I am committed to healthy living, because God lovingly assures me that I am worthy of this and even more.

"Look at the birds of the air; they neither sow nor reap nor gather into barns, and yet your heavenly Father feeds them. Are you not of more value than they?"
—Matthew 6:26

TODAY'S MESSAGE

Look at Me

I look at myself and rejoice that I am a new person.

Look at me: I feel comfortable being in the first row of a group of people being photographed. Not that I am showing off; I simply no longer feel the need to hide behind others.

Look at how I walk and move: I have a spring in my step and a smoothness of movement. I feel good about how much more easily I can bend down.

When I look at myself, I see less of me, but by getting rid of extra weight, I have relieved my heart and joints. I am not the person I was a few weeks ago; I am in better health and have greater peace of mind.

I have known all along that God accepts and loves me as I was and as I am, but I am feeling so much better about myself now. Feeling good physically and emotionally, I find so much to love about myself and others.

"Father, I desire that those also, whom you have given me, may be with me where I am, to see my glory, which you have given me because you loved me before the foundation of the world."
—John 17:24

Today's Message

Bright Future

***Living in the moments of today,
I am building a bright future for my tomorrows.***

I still may be holding on to an image of myself the way I was before I lost weight. Then when I catch a glimpse of my reflection in a store window or actually study my reflection in a mirror, I realize how much I have changed. My clothes fit better now, and I feel more energetic.

I have changed not only my appearance but also the way I think, eat, and live my life. I am living in the bright future that I envisioned months before, and I am glad I kept on track by taking responsibility for eating nutritious food and devoting time to physical activity.

And I keep on this positive track. I can only live in the now of today, but my positive thoughts and actions are helping me create a bright future in which I will enjoy the results of the good thoughts and habits I have expressed in the past.

**"My child, eat honey, for it is good. . . .
Know that wisdom is such to your soul;
if you find it, you will find a future."
—Proverbs 24:13–14**

Today's Message

For a Lifetime

I honor the gift of life by treating myself with care and reverence for a lifetime.

I have often heard the saying, "I am eating to live, not living to eat." I know that as I eat to live, wonderful results emerge: As I make selections in right proportions from the different food groups, I lose weight—a pound or two a week. I discover how to not only lose weight but to also eat for a lifetime of health and well-being.

God has given me life, and I am dedicated to honoring the gift of life by treating it with care and reverence every day. With good nutrition and frequent exercise, strength building activity, and daily prayer, I am honoring the gift of life. And I am dedicated to doing all these things and even more for a lifetime.

The habits and practices that I follow consistently for a month or so become a part of my routine. And my health-promoting routine becomes a part of my life—for a lifetime.

"Those who drink of the water that I will give them will never be thirsty. The water that I will give will become in them a spring of water gushing up to eternal life."
—John 4:14

Meditation

I Am More

God's spirit within me encourages me to be more and provides me with all I need to be more.

God, I come to You in this sacred time of prayer for assurance. I tune out all distractions around me and give my full attention to You.

"Beloved, put aside all doubt and know that you can do anything you set your mind and heart on doing. You are more than you are aware of being.

"Now think on this: You are life and love and wisdom being expressed through a mind and body. Yet you are more, for My spirit resides within you.

"You are more than a person who lives for a certain number of years. You are an eternal being that can never be separated from Me.

"Rest now, beloved, and know that I am a presence within you that is encouraging you and providing all that you will need to be more."

"And God is able to provide you with every blessing in abundance, so that by always having enough of everything, you may share abundantly in every good work."
—2 Corinthians 9:8

◆ *Journal* ◆

Date: ______________________________

My weight: __________________________

I make the most of what this day has to offer and live my life to the fullest.

I can ______________________________

Today's Message

Needed and Important

Knowing that I am needed and important to God, I live in a way that expresses my divine nature.

How do I know that I am needed and important? Perhaps I have family members who depend on my loving care. My coworkers may count on my enthusiasm and good ideas.

There are countless other ways in which I am needed, but most significant is this: I am important to God! I am the hands by which God touches another life. I am the words through which God comforts someone or the voice whose song uplifts another person.

Of this I am certain: I have a place in the world that only I can fill. I have a true sense of importance and purpose. My purpose is to live in a way that most fully expresses my divine nature. I do this by being loving, compassionate, and kind to others and to myself.

Whatever I choose to do and however I express myself, I know that I am fulfilling my divine purpose. I am needed and important.

"God saw everything that he had made, and indeed, it was very good."
—Genesis 1:31

Today's Message

Patience

Being patient with myself and my progress, I encourage myself to make greater progress.

Realizing how much I have accomplished is gratifying. If after a while the progress is not as dramatic, I may feel impatient with myself. But I remain true to my dedication because I know that my new healthy way of life is blessing me. Even if my shape does not show a remarkable reduction in size, I remember that, inside me, each cell is constantly being energized and renewed by a healthy balance of nutritious food and exercise.

By taking my time and remaining patient with myself, I avoid the pitfalls of yo-yo dieting. I follow my doctor's instructions, partnered with life-affirming prayers and times of quiet meditation. If I am happy with these techniques, I continue with them. If not, I have patience with myself and faith in God to guide me to a better weight-management program.

"Keep on doing the things that you have learned and received and heard and seen in me, and the God of peace will be with you."
—Philippians 4:9

Today's Message

Ready and Willing

I am ready and willing to love and to be loved.

Before I can accept and truly appreciate the love and understanding of others, I must first love myself. Feeling good about myself, I feel at peace.

I am ready and willing to love myself and appreciate all that I have accomplished and am capable of achieving. I respect myself and recognize the wonderful potential that is within me.

When I look in the mirror, I see a remarkable person worthy of God's love and open and receptive to the love of others. In my prayers I bless myself as well as all those that I am praying for.

Creating an atmosphere of love within and around me, I continue to learn about myself and to treat myself with kindness and consideration. I radiate love.

I am ready and willing to be blessed by love and to bless others with love.

"As God's chosen ones, holy and beloved, clothe yourselves with compassion, kindness, humility, meekness, and patience."
—Colossians 3:12

Today's Message

Positive Approach

I congratulate myself for what I have achieved, and with a positive approach, I expect continued success.

The ways I eat and exercise have changed for the better. But even with the best of intentions, there may be times when I overindulge by eating a large portion of a rich dessert or I declare that I don't have time to exercise because of a busy schedule. Rather than berate myself, I remind myself that I have been successful in losing the weight, and each day I am continually making strides in maintaining my weight.

A few months or even a year of following a weight-loss plan can be considered a short-term project—considering the years that are before me. Maintaining my optimal weight is a long-term, lifelong commitment of investing in myself.

What I have done so far has been no small feat, and I congratulate myself for what I have achieved. With a positive approach, I expect continued success.

"The Lord bless you and keep you; the Lord make his face to shine upon you, and be gracious to you; the Lord lift up his countenance upon you, and give you peace."
—Numbers 6:24–26

Today's Message

Individuality

God's is the wisdom and guidance I follow in expressing my individuality.

I am a unique individual, and only God and I know what is right and true for me. With God's help, I am continuing to transform myself into the healthier, more fit person I would like to be. By working in cooperation with God, I am growing increasingly more aware of my spiritual heritage of health.

At this point, I am fully aware of which diet and exercise techniques have produced good results, and it has been with great delight that I have seen the numbers on the scale going down. Now I concentrate on keeping the weight off. Again my approach to this is as individual as I am.

I am interested in what others offer as advice or share as helpful tips, and I thank them for their thoughtfulness. My focus remains on my own individuality and the assurance that God is directing me so that my unique needs are met.

"But you are not in the flesh; you are in the Spirit, since the Spirit of God dwells in you."
—Romans 8:9

Today's Message

What's Next?

I look forward to the future with eager anticipation.

I may find that with the changes in my body, my outlook on life has gradually been changing as well. I feel more energized and enthusiastic throughout the day, and I keep a positive outlook, even during times that would have been stressful for me in the past.

With this new attitude, I may also begin to question what is next for me since I have already met my goals.

When I ponder "What's next?" in my life, I remain calm and collected, for I know that wherever I may go, whatever I may do, God goes with me and before me. I look forward to the future with eager anticipation.

My goals may change, but one thing is for certain: God will always remain the same—a constant, loving presence in my life.

"Therefore I tell you, do not worry about your life, what you will eat, or about your body, what you will wear. For life is more than food, and the body more than clothing."
—Luke 12:22–23

MEDITATION

New Creation

As I rest in silence, I feel God's presence empowering me. I am a new creation!

I rest in the silence with God, considering the new creation that I am as I near and even reach my weight-loss goal.

Gently, thankfully, I close my eyes and in my mind's eye, I behold the new creation that I am. I offer words of positive reinforcement and wisdom to myself. Then I give thanks to God:

"I am thankful that I took the necessary steps in taking control of my thoughts and actions, which are powerfully reflected in my body now.

"I thank You, God, for blessing me along my journey. I am at peace with the changes that I have made—changes that lead to a new, trimmer me. I appreciate who I am and all that You are to me."

As I rest in silence, I feel God's presence empowering me. I am a new creation!

**"Every day I will bless you,
and praise your name forever and ever."
—Psalms 145:2**

◆ *Journal* ◆

Date: ____

My weight: ___________________________________

I can be a source of encouragement
for others who may be trying
to lose weight.

My words of wisdom would include ________

____

____

____

____

____

____

____

____

____

____

A positive attitude seems to make things easier to deal with by making problems seem smaller than they really are. You can change your attitude by viewing your life in positive tones. . . . Just look for the good and watch your songs of anger transform into tunes of happiness and love.

◆

Source: Recipes for Life *by Edie Hand*

A New Self-Image

By Peggy Pifer

For much of my adult life, my weight has been a sensitive subject for me, and putting into words my experience with weight loss is not an easy thing to do. I don't continually analyze my life experiences and myself in order to determine what led me to gain weight, even though I am becoming more aware of those reasons and dealing with those issues. I concentrate on what I can do to take corrective action now.

There are many methods and programs that help different individuals lose weight. I know that, for many people, strict diets are helpful, and many people have been quite successful while using them. Personally, I have not had much success with diets that restrict me to only a few choices. They become too expensive or so boring that I cannot follow them for long, which may be the same result for many others.

I believe that each individual has to discover the method that works best for her or him, and as with any lifestyle change, each individual has to be ready to make a commitment to maintaining that change.

Sometimes a simple realization can be the key to unlocking the door to successful weight loss. I had such a realization about a year ago that should have seemed

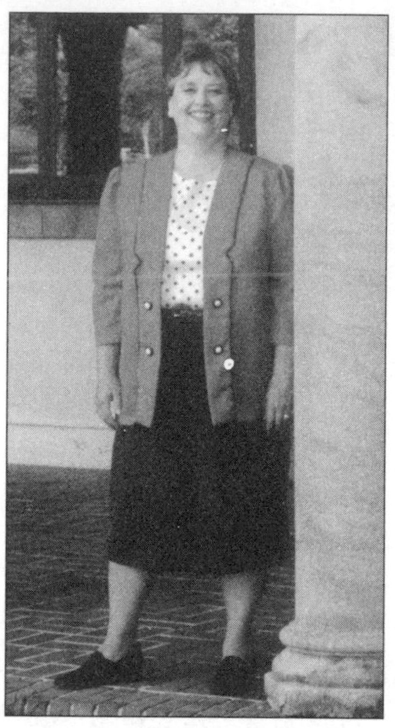

obvious to me a long time before: I could not eat the way my tall, slender husband eats and not gain weight. His metabolism is much different than mine, and at his very physical job he burns up lots of calories every day. I enjoy the food I plan and cook for him as much as, and probably more than, he does. For 25 years I ate like he did. You wouldn't think it would take me so long to figure it out, but what is important is that I did.

I had reached a point where I felt tired and anxious. I was not sleeping well, and my energy level was low. I knew I had to make a change. Because a specific diet menu had never worked well for me, I decided to adopt a general plan that combined healthy eating and brisk walking. I included more fruits, vegetables, and whole grain food in my diet. I ate less fat and no sugar. For the first time in my life, I didn't feel as though I was on a difficult diet. I felt good. I started slowly, first cutting back on food in the evening—nothing to eat after 7:30 P.M. For an in-between meal treat, I ate a cup of orange juice or skim milk (with a few drops of vanilla added) that had been in the freezer just long enough to be at a thickened, slushy consistency. Or I ate a sugar-free popsicle that satisfied my craving for dessert.

I also spent time meditating, praying, and blessing my body. I gave thanks to God for the wisdom within me that guided my decisions and for the presence of life within that kept my body in good working order.

The weight slowly came off—35 pounds in a year's time—and I managed to keep it off for a year and a half.

Something unexpected happened after the weight loss: Although losing weight had changed my appearance, the image I had of myself had remained the same. I still thought of myself as being the size I was 35 pounds heavier. Even though I had obviously lost weight (the scales do not lie) and was wearing smaller sizes, I did not think of myself as a smaller person. Granted, I still had more weight to lose, but somehow, I still held a mental picture of my former self, not my new, slimmer self.

People were very generous with their compliments. Coworkers who knew me well and even some who did not remarked on my weight loss. Even with their encouraging words, I was still surprised when I was able to fit into clothes I had not worn in a long time or when I suddenly discovered I could shop in the "Misses" section instead of the "Women's" section of the clothing store.

It is funny when I think back about it. I was always surprised when I found something in the back of my closet that I could wear. It did not dawn on me that the reason it was there was because it had been too tight and uncomfortable for me to wear. For all intents and purposes, it seemed as if I was trying to deny that I was succeeding.

The way everyone else saw me was not the way I saw myself. Even though I could wear clothes I had not worn for a long time, even though I was buying new clothes in a smaller size, I did not think of myself as being any smaller. As a matter of fact, I have one persistent friend who told me more than once that I should not wear one particular pair of slacks again because they were too big. I even argued with her! But she insisted, and finally I gave in and stopped wearing them. Everyone needs a friend like this! Still, I left the pants hanging in my closet for months before I had the courage, or maybe the understanding, to get rid of them.

But one day I had somewhat of an "Aha" moment when I tried on an outfit that my daughter had given me for my birthday the previous year. I had put it aside because even though I had managed to get the slacks on and zipped and the top buttoned, they were both too tight. When I tried the outfit on a year later, the slacks were much more comfortable, and the top was so loose that I could grab a handful of extra material. I was amazed and began to adjust my self-image to fit the slimmer me.

I have not completely solved my image problem. And I do want to lose more weight. As a matter of fact, I gained some weight, but I am happy to say that I am back on track again. I know that along with eating right and exercising, I also need to work on my self-image in order to make further progress.

A positive self-image means so much. How I see myself and how others see me may be very different. Even if I am a kind and compassionate person with others, I can be hard on myself, critical of the way I look. To help me improve the inner picture I have of myself, I practice seeing myself in a more positive light. I praise myself for every accomplishment, no matter how small it may appear. When I avoid eating calorie-loaded food, I give myself a pat on the back. For every meal at which I eat only healthy foods, for every bit of weight I lose, I remember to congratulate myself for keeping my commitment to lose weight and for my success in losing it. For every task I complete, I remember to tell myself, "Well done!"

These are some other things I am doing to raise my self-image:

I write down my strong points—what I like and appreciate about myself.

I read my list and add to it regularly

I listen—with gratitude—to the good things people tell me about myself.

Most important, I remember that—because I am one of my Creator's creations, made in God's image and likeness—I am a spiritual being. So I know that looking within my soul, I will find my true self, a spiritual being that is whole in every way. This is the true part of me that I speak about when I affirm: *I am strong, for I have strength of Spirit.* I know that this is the truth about myself, for I have the strength of God within me. With this strength, I am able to resist the temptation to eat food that my body does not need or is not nourished by. When I feel the urge to reach for a cookie or some potato chips, I take just a moment to remember my true self and know that I am strong enough to make choices that benefit my well-being.

I know the truth about myself as I affirm in thought, word, and action the picture of what I want to look like: the healthy me who has achieved my goal. I do this by affirming the truth about myself and giving thanks for this truth even before I see the complete outcome: *I am healthy, and I give thanks to God for guiding me so that I achieve the weight that is right for me.*

If I do experience a lapse in my commitment, I do not view myself as having failed. As a spiritual being, I do not believe in defeat. I encourage myself to begin again right where I am.

Knowing that I am a spiritual being, filled with the strength and wisdom of God, I continue to make progress!

Today's Message

Good Enough

With all that I am and all that I do as God's creation, I am good enough for the very best in life!

I may have discovered that as my weight increased, my self-esteem decreased. I did not feel good enough the way I was. Now that I look and feel better, I have greater confidence. Yet I realize that my weight—now or in the past—does not define who I am. As God's creation, I have always been and will always be good enough!

I am good enough to try for my dream job. I have been building self-confidence and skills that now qualify me for my chosen profession. I am able to do what this job requires me to do and capable of learning even more.

I am good enough to expect and accept the best of all that life has to offer me. I am a fantastic blend of spirit, mind, and body—a divine creation living a human experience, and I do so with grace and love.

Yes, I am ready to fulfill my heart's desire.

"May the Lord direct your hearts to the love of God and to the steadfastness of Christ."
—2 Thessalonians 3:5

Today's Message
New Wardrobe

—◆—

I sparkle with a joy of Spirit that transforms me.

There is so much more to me than what others see, yet I want to look my best because it is a reflection of how good I feel about myself. I may not look like a model, because that is not me.

However, this may be the time for me to buy a new pair of jeans or a new swimsuit. Do I even know my current size? I may have a pleasant surprise awaiting me as I try on clothes.

If I checked my closet now, would I see a rack of dark clothes? Then I may include some bright colors in my new wardrobe. The brightness of my clothes helps brighten my outlook. Shopping is once again a fun activity!

I look different on the outside, but something else is different about me. The most important element of the new me comes from within: Clothed in the joy of Spirit, I sparkle with life.

"You have turned my mourning into dancing, you have taken off my sackcloth and clothed me with joy." —Psalms 30:11

TODAY'S MESSAGE

Being Objective

God shines the light of truth on my path.

Something as unfavorable as a weight gain of a pound or two may stop me in my tracks. That is when I may question, "Whoa! Wait a minute—why is this happening to me?"

Then I can do one of two things—I remain at a standstill while I search for someone or something to blame or I take positive steps forward and move on. I choose to take the positive approach of a divine path.

I turn my attention to God, quiet my mind, and ask for the wisdom and guidance that enable me to attain a view of my life from a higher, more objective perspective.

God shines the light of truth on my thoughts, and I am able to see that there is a clear way ahead of me. When I perceive my life from this spiritual outlook, I see the divine path before me and I move forward along it.

**"O send out your light and your truth;
let them lead me; let them bring me to your holy hill
and to your dwelling."
—Psalms 43:3**

Today's Message

Seeds of Wisdom

Seeds of divine wisdom bring renewed hope and joy into my life.

When I read or hear something that speaks to my heart on an intimate level, I have an "Aha" moment— a surge of inspiration that brings an undeniable clarity to my thoughts. Seeds of divine wisdom are creative thoughts that have been planted in the fertile soil of my mind. I nourish these ideas so that they grow and flourish. The spirit of God encourages me to use my imagination and creativity to express divine ideas.

Such encouragement may come as I am riding in my car, listening to the radio. A favorite song is played, and I sense a surge of joy and feel uplifted. I may read someone's true-life story and be so inspired by this person's experience that my thoughts are: Yes! That is exactly how I felt. Yet I couldn't seem to find the right words to express it to others.

I am grateful for seeds of divine wisdom that bring renewed hope and joy into my life at just the right moment that I need them.

"I planted, Apollos watered, but God gave the growth."
—1 Corinthians 3:6

Today's Message

Creative Person

Destined by God to be a creative person,
I can be successful in whatever I say and do.

God has already prepared me to be all that I was created to be. I am perfectly capable of reaching my ideal weight and learning to maintain it, so I pay attention to what I eat and how active I am.

If I feel myself slipping into old habits of overeating and inactivity, I look for creative ways to boost my morale and stay interested in maintaining my weight. A picture of the way I looked months ago and one of how I look now may help me stay focused on my success. Modifying old recipes, trying new recipes, or choosing new foods benefit me and my family. Keeping a favorite craft project close by, working in my garden, or visiting with friends or neighbors eases the way through boredom, loneliness, and fatigue.

In my daily prayer, I thank God for preparing the way for me and guiding me in doing what is best.

"For we are what he has made us, created in Christ Jesus for good works, which God prepared beforehand to be our way of life."
—Ephesians 2:10

Today's Message

Breathe

—◆—

My deep, steady breathing focuses me on the peace of God within, and I am calm.

Something as simple as basic breathing is an action plan that takes me from feeling stressed to being calm. And when I am calm, I make wise decisions.

If I should experience symptoms of anxiety—accelerated heart rate, shortness of breath, uneasiness—I take a moment to settle into a chair, close my eyes, and take a slow, deep breath that fills my lungs to capacity.

Then I begin to slowly exhale. As the air gently leaves my body, tension fades with it, and I relax. Continuing my deep-breathing exercise, I encourage my heart rate to return to normal. My breathing focuses my thoughts on the peace of God within me, and I remain in that peaceful realm for several minutes. Thoughts of stress are gone and peaceful thoughts thrive. My exercise in breathing has heightened my awareness of divine life within me.

**"I will greatly rejoice in the Lord,
my whole being shall exult in my God."
—Isaiah 61:10**

MEDITATION
In the Light

Basking in the light of God,
I give thanks to my Creator.

I feel every shadow of doubt receding as—alone with God—I acknowledge my Creator's loving presence. All darkness gives way to light, a brilliant light that guides my way. In thanksgiving to God, I express my appreciation:

"In Your presence, dear God, I feel like a flower that is unfolding in the bright light of day, growing within the warm environment of Your love and wisdom. And like that flower, I continue to reveal bloom after bloom of joy and love.

"In Your light, God, I find new ways to share Your message of hope and love with others. Thank You, God, for lighting my way and for revealing the blessings that are before me. Because of You and with You, I am growing and learning."

"He led them in safety,
so that they were not afraid."
—Psalms 78:53

◆ *Journal* ◆

Date: ______________________________

My weight: __________________________

I am investing in my future
through healthy living.

As I consider the future, I see myself ________

____

____

____

____

____

____

____

____

____

____

Today's Message

Support

—◆—

God supports me—
unconditionally and eternally.

God is my constant source of support. In any moment of doubt or with even a thought of giving up on myself, I hear a whisper of assurance from God. This is an assurance that my soul hears and responds to. In a quiet moment of rest, God is the silence that fills my mind with peace.

God knows that I am doing my best—according to my understanding of what is best. My Creator has faith in me—a faith that encourages me to enhance my understanding and to learn from all of my experiences.

In every moment of the day and night, God sustains me—unconditionally and without fail. Knowing that the love of God upholds me now and throughout all time fills me with peace and reassurance.

"Where you go, I will go; where you lodge,
I will lodge; your people shall be my people,
and your God my God."
—Ruth 1:16

TODAY'S MESSAGE

Starting Over

Open to my goodness, I invite blessings into my life, and I accept them with gratitude to God.

Realistically, I am starting over with each new day that dawns. So I know not to become discouraged when I don't meet my own expectations of what I am able to achieve on any certain day or by any certain number of months.

But when I do overeat or skip exercising, I go back to my original commitment and start over. I know better than to sabotage my efforts by letting one meal or one day of overeating lead to another.

God gives me spiritual insight and energy that enable me to rise above any lapses in my healthy behavior. Right now I break the link of misbehaving that would lead to a weight gain. How good it is to be in control. I am starting over by doing things that are good for me. Open to my goodness, I invite blessings into my life, and I accept them with gratitude.

"The Lord will guide you continually, and satisfy your needs in parched places, and make your bones strong; and you shall be like a watered garden."
—Isaiah 58:11

Today's Message

Taking Care

Divine life within me responds to my prayers with healing energy.

God created me, and it is to God that I turn when I need help taking care of myself. In considering my health and well-being, I remember that God and I work together as a team.

God has designed an intricate system of tissue and nerves within my body that lets me know when something is not quite right and may need attention. Having listened to what my body was telling me, I then give my undivided attention to God, using prayer as a means of responding in a caring way.

If there is pain in any part of my body, I close my eyes and begin to bless the pain away by visualizing the healing power that is released in prayer. Divine life within me responds. A powerful force of energy moves throughout my body, renewing and recharging every cell with life.

"In his hand is the life of every living thing and the breath of every human being."
—Job 12:10

TODAY'S MESSAGE

New Discoveries

—◆—

God directs my steps and leads me daily on a path of discovering new skills and strengths.

Each day I make new discoveries about how wonderful it is to be at a healthy weight. Each day I discover how easy some tasks are now that were difficult or impossible for me in the past. Each day brings a new awareness of how I can manage my weight when I trust God for wisdom and guidance.

I look and feel like a new person who has positive feelings and a positive attitude toward myself and others. As I continue to be in control of my eating habits, I feel better both physically and emotionally. I discover new reserves of energy and new tastes in food. I have the ability to distinguish between what I think I *want* and what I *need* to stay healthy.

When my weight-loss plans are interrupted, I trust God to direct my thoughts and actions so that I stay true to my purpose. With confidence, I continue to discover new ways of maintaining my weight.

"The human mind plans the way, but the Lord directs the steps."
—Proverbs 16:9

TODAY'S MESSAGE

My Teachers

—◆—

I am grateful for the love, dedication, and faith of all those who have taught me.

Many different people have been my teachers—not only the ones who instructed me in school but also teachers in life as well. These are people who loved me, cared for me, and wanted only the best for me.

My teachers have been parents, siblings, grandparents, and friends who taught me about how great it is to love and understand one another.

My ultimate teacher is God—the One from whom I receive love and guidance in their purest forms and with my unique needs in mind. My Creator is wisdom that surpasses the ages and is the one true source of knowledge. God not only provides for me, but teaches me the life skills I need to make my way easier. In my relationship with God, I receive the courage to persevere, the love and understanding to accept all people as family, and the gentleness to embrace the beauty and majesty that surround me.

"Lead me in your truth, and teach me,
for you are the God of my salvation."
—Psalms 25:5

Today's Message

A Matter of Choice

—◆—

Every day God gives me a fresh 24 hours in which to make choices that enrich my life.

Every day is a composite of the choices I make and the choices of others that impact my life. I cannot control others, but I am always adding to and taking away from my day with the decisions I make.

Having made the choice to weigh less and sticking with my choice, I have lost weight. And it is my choice to live as that thinner, healthier person I have become. I renew that choice every day, because I know how important it is to me.

By the grace of God, I am given the chance to make choices every day. I am learning to make ones that enrich my life. My self-confidence grows as my weight continues to go down and then stabilizes. Each new day is awaiting my consideration of what will add meaning and purpose to my life, and my choices are divinely guided ones that bless me.

"According to the grace of God given to me, like a skilled master builder I laid a foundation, and someone else is building on it. Each builder must choose with care how to build on it."
—1 Corinthians 3:10

MEDITATION

Before and After

Fulfilled by who I am and how much I have accomplished, I savor the present moment with God.

I relax, knowing that I am in the presence of God. Letting all worry and concern melt away, I speak to God of how far I have come and how much further I can go with my Creator's help:

"God, as I relax for a few moments with You, I leave behind the past and savor the present moment. I have come a long way with my dedication to being healthier and more fulfilled. There has been a change in me.

"I think about the feeling of satisfaction that spreads over me when others noticed my accomplishments. I feel even better right now because I know that You have been aware of each hurdle I have overcome, which has brought me to what is visibly evident now. There is a before and after of me, God, but You have been my support all the while."

"And while he was praying, the appearance of his face changed, and his clothes became dazzling white."
—Luke 9:29

◆ *Journal* ◆

Date: ________________________________

My weight: ____________________________

This is an extraordinary day,
and I thank God
for every moment of it.

I thank God for ________________________

____

____

____

____

____

____

____

____

____

____

Today's Message

Taking a Break

I take a break from the activities of my day to experience God's presence.

Before I realize what is happening, I can become caught up in the "busyness" of my day. So when I start to feel rushed or on overload, I take a break and treat myself to a moment of quiet reflection.

I may also feel the need to take a break from my diet and treat myself to something special. A treat may be a once-a-week reward for keeping myself healthy and working toward my goal.

Today, I may take several breaks and for a few moments sit quietly. Taking a break and relaxing for a while is important, for in this tranquil time, I experience the peace of God's presence within and around me.

This is a God break that gives me strength of mind and body—a strength that enables me to continue the activities of the day feeling refreshed and rewarded.

**"O taste and see that the Lord is good;
happy are those who take refuge in him."
—Psalms 34:8**

TODAY'S MESSAGE

Being Fit

—◆—

Through the power of God's spirit within me, I am physically fit and able to be active over a lifetime.

My purpose in establishing better eating and exercise habits is not only to reach a greater level of fitness but also to retain that level and even move past it. To do this, I express determination, courage, and dedication every day.

I can because I recognize that I have spiritual power within that upholds me in reaching and maintaining a quality of physical fitness that allows me to be active over a lifetime.

If I were able to hear the response of my body to what I have achieved, I believe this is what I would hear: My heart would say, "Thank you for not giving up and for keeping up." And my bones and joints would say, "We are so relieved and grateful!"

I am strong and courageous, because the spirit of God is living within me and out through me as determination, courage, and dedication to success.

"Be strong, and let your heart take courage, all you who wait for the Lord."
—Psalms 31:24

Today's Message

Time Management

I manage my time by planning for accomplishment and enjoyment.

An inner voice of intuition is quick to remind me that I may not have time enough in one day to finish everything that I would like. Yet when I do plan ahead for my day, I prioritize. And prioritizing helps me balance what I *need* to do with what I would *like* to do. I then manage my time, and I am able to enjoy my day.

As I use time management to organize, I use my time wisely and efficiently. Gone is the hurried feeling that I experienced when I suddenly remembered an appointment at the last minute. Gone is the sensation of being overwhelmed with things to do around my home.

Considering my schedule, I may include time for reading a lighthearted book for the purpose of being entertained. I may decide to see the movie that showed so much promise in a preview I saw weeks ago. I make time and I take the time to do those things I *wish* to do much more than *need* to do.

**"The uneven ground shall become level,
and the rough places a plain."
—Isaiah 40:4**

Today's Message

Consistency

Being consistent in my faith, I am consistent in holding on to my weight loss.

I have been inspired by other peoples' stories of weight loss. I have picked up helpful tips that worked well for me. I have been encouraged because I understood that if it was possible for them to lose weight, I could also.

There are many more untold success stories of people that I meet every day. I may see a thin woman and never know that she has lost 50 pounds and kept it off for 10 years! Yet when I hear her story, I probably will learn that she has been consistent in her approach to staying thin. What she eats and the way she eats have not fluctuated drastically over the years and neither has her weight.

I comprehend a faith and strength in others that I emulate myself. Being consistent in my faith and weight, I am inspired and I inspire others to do the same.

"Remember your leaders, those who spoke the word of God to you; consider the outcome of their way of life, and imitate their faith. Jesus Christ is the same yesterday and today and forever."
—Hebrews 13:7–8

Today's Message

Embracing Life

I embrace life with an enthusiasm for exploring God's creativity.

There are times when I need to cheer myself up. And there are times I also cheer myself on in recognizing what I have achieved and believing that I can do even more.

Even in the toughest situation, I learn something of value. For instance, I may feel discouraged about a misunderstanding with someone, but I do not turn to food for solace as I have in the past. I turn to God and am comforted and lead to a way that I can help resolve the matter.

Because I embrace life with enthusiasm, I accept that the ups and downs of life are part of the process of me becoming wiser and more self-confident. I am eager to explore the wonder of God in my world and to give thanks for how much God blesses me.

By embracing life as an outpouring of God's creativity and love, I open my eyes and my soul to the abundance of God that is everywhere.

"Do not lag in zeal, be ardent in spirit, serve the Lord."
—Romans 12:11

Today's Message

A Dream Come True

—◆—

With God to guide me, I follow my dreams, and my dreams really do come true.

As a child, I may have been prone to daydreaming—imagining how my life would unfold and wondering what, if any, great achievements I would make. Over time I matured, and my dreams altered as my priorities in life changed.

One dream of being a thinner, healthier person may have surpassed all others of my hopeful imaginings. Now that I am able to maintain my weight loss, I feel a sense of accomplishment, and I celebrate a dream that has come true.

My dream is now a reality, and I congratulate myself by buying a new outfit or taking a day off from work just to pamper myself. My self-confidence has been strengthened, and my life has been enriched by a dream come true.

"Then the Lord came down in a pillar of cloud, and stood at the entrance of the tent. . . . And he said, 'Hear my words: . . . I the Lord make myself known to them in visions; I speak to them in dreams.'"
—Numbers 12:5–6

MEDITATION

Honoring My Progress

God honors my progress by supporting me and encouraging me.

Moving in thought to the quiet recesses of my soul, I congratulate myself for all that I have accomplished. It is here in the silence that God whispers words of encouragement to me and support for the progress I have made:

"My child, you have made tremendous strides in your journey. I know it has not been an easy road for you, but I trust you have felt My presence with you every step of the way.

"You have learned not to allow your emotions to interfere with your good judgment. When you felt upset, you sought peace through Me rather than comfort through food.

"As you continue your journey, I will be with you—to guide you, to comfort you, to support you, to laugh with you, to love you through it all."

"When we cry, 'Abba! Father!' it is that very Spirit bearing witness with our spirit that we are children of God."
—Romans 8:15–16

◆ *Journal* ◆

Date: ________________________________

My weight: ____________________________

Just as I nourish my body
with healthy foods, I nourish my soul
through my times of prayer and meditation.

Today my prayers include ________________

____

____

____

____

____

____

____

____

____

____

TODAY'S MESSAGE

Feeling Good

—◆—

I feel good!

I feel good today! What an amazing transformation is taking place within me—mentally, physically, and spiritually.

I breathe easier. Where before I may not have felt inclined to take part in much physical activity, I find that now I can walk farther and climb stairs more easily.

I have more energy. I want to do more, to get out and about more. The projects I have been delaying no longer seem to be overwhelming. With new strength and vigor, I am ready to do those things that I previously procrastinated doing.

I walk with new energy and enthusiasm, with a new sense of confidence in myself, because with the help of God, I have accomplished wonderful goals.

I am ready for new adventures. I know there is so much more that I can do, and as I set new goals, I trust God to show me the way to their fulfillment.

"A glad heart makes a cheerful countenance."
—Proverbs 15:13

Today's Message
Next Horizon

I keep my sights set on the heights—the greater good of God that is awaiting me.

Taking a journey by car, I have a unique opportunity to see the horizon ahead. Mile after mile, the scene changes as horizon after horizon comes into view.

Life can seem like a journey that takes me from one hill or mountain top to the next. Having finally reached a point of a former horizon, I have still another destination to reach in a horizon miles ahead.

At these times, I lift my vision from the depths of the valley and keep my sights set on the heights—the greater good that God has for me.

If I need help, I know that it is always available, for God is with me throughout my life's journey. Looking to God keeps me focused on the true source of every blessing that I receive and every blessing that lies ahead, awaiting me.

"I will lift up my eyes to the hills—
from where will my help come?
My help comes from the Lord,
who made heaven and earth."
—Psalms 121:1–2

TODAY'S MESSAGE

Reimage

Thank You, God, for helping me see my new image—a successful, happy, healthy person.

A photograph is an image of what the camera lens "sees." The photographer can produce different images by changing the focus of the lens or by focusing the lens on different subjects.

With my mind's eye, I see an image of myself. Like the photographer, I can change this image by changing my focus: the way I direct my thoughts.

When I consider the progress I have made in losing weight, I think that perhaps it is time to take another look at this image I hold of myself. In the past I may have held a negative image. Right now is a good time to "reimage" myself and improve my self-image. Quiet times with God will help me do this, for God will help me change my focus, so that I see my good qualities. I can begin to see myself as the successful, happy, healthy person that God created me to be.

"And all of us, with unveiled faces, seeing the glory of the Lord as though reflected in a mirror, are being transformed into the same image from one degree of glory to another."
—2 Corinthians 3:18

TODAY'S MESSAGE

Extraordinary Day

This is an extraordinary day, and I express my enthusiasm and appreciation for it.

How I may yearn for something special to do or to happen today. Because I know that boredom led me to overeat in the past, I don't want to become bored, and even if I do, I don't want that to cause me to overeat!

When I stop to think about my day, however, I understand that the people and things that I tend to take for granted are what actually make my day special and extraordinary. Holding a child in my arms and feeling the soft, tender skin against mine; being joyously greeted by my pet when I come home at the end of the day; hearing a loved one say, "I love you!" all make my spirits soar.

There is no day that is routine when I include communion with God in that day. The spiritual connection I realize infuses me with both enthusiasm for and appreciation of life and all the experiences of my day—every day.

"Great is our Lord, and abundant in power; his understanding is beyond measure."
—Psalms 147:5

Today's Message

Countdown

Counting my successes, I feel happy, confident, and successful.

For the past few months, I have concentrated my time and energy on the specific goal of losing weight. I may have set a target date and completed my goal. Counting down to this date taught me the value of staying focused and of keeping my thoughts positive—traits that I can use for any goal I set my mind and heart to accomplish.

Keeping a count of the pounds I have lost and seeing results come about have certainly been fulfilling experiences, but the most fulfilling aspects of my weight-loss program are the things I have learned about myself and the confidence I have gained. Through my commitment, I have become a more positive and focused individual.

I give thanks for the new person I have become. I know that I am divinely guided and that I can do whatever is important to my health and well-being.

"I cry to God Most High, to God who fulfills his purpose for me."
—Psalms 57:2

Today's Message

Rainy Days

***Uplifting my thoughts,
I make the best of what this day offers me.***

Children who are playing outside sense they are in the midst of God's creation. They play in and with the wind, grass, and leaves. Their laughter joins in with the songs of birds. On rainy days, however, children use their imaginations to create their own fun world. They play and laugh and fill houses and schoolrooms with the sunshine of their exhilaration.

What do I do on gray days when I feel a bit down? I too use my imagination and creativity to let sunshine into my life. I am a child of God, and my Creator has given me a mind, spirit, and body to do with as I will. And I will do my very best to honor God by taking care of myself.

Whenever gray clouds appear, I know the sun will shine again and there will be a rainbow, a promise of better times.

**"When I bring clouds over the earth and the bow is seen in the clouds, I will remember my covenant that is between me and you and every living creature."
—Genesis 9:14**

MEDITATION

Freedom to Be

God has given me the freedom to be whatever I dedicate myself to being.

At times in the past, I have used my being overweight as an excuse not to step beyond my usual comfort zone and dare to try something new.

Today, in a time of sacred meditation, I renew my commitment to be free of limitation.

Relaxed and still, I picture this scene: There is a thinner me moving past the heavy image of what I used to be. I have a smile on my face, because I realize that I am free to make new discoveries about my talents and abilities. Thankful to God for love and support, I realize I want to try to do whatever brings me the greatest fulfillment and meaning in life. Yes, I have the freedom to be whatever I dedicate myself to being.

I know beyond a doubt that the wisdom of God guides me and the love of God reassures me. I rest in the awareness of my freedom to be.

"When Jesus saw her, he called her over and said, 'Woman, you are set free from your ailment.'"
—Luke 13:12

◆ *Journal* ◆

Date: ______________________________

My weight: __________________________

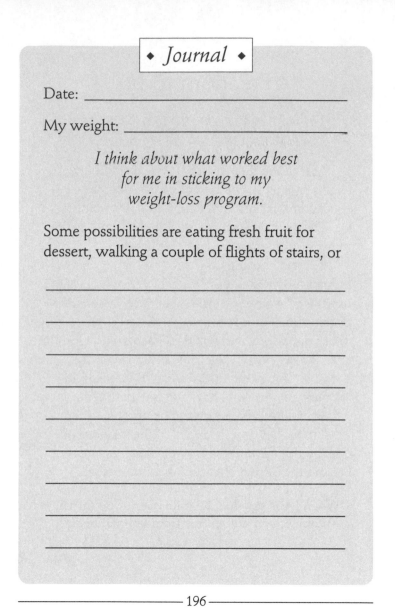

I think about what worked best for me in sticking to my weight-loss program.

Some possibilities are eating fresh fruit for dessert, walking a couple of flights of stairs, or

____

____

____

____

____

____

____

____

____

When reading food labels, keep in mind the following terms as defined by the Food and Drug Administration (FDA):

Calorie-free *means fewer than 5 calories per serving.*

Low calorie *means 40 calories or less per serving.*

Sugar-free *or* fat-free *both mean less than 0.5 grams per serving.*

◆

Honoring My Contract with God
By Kat Carney

When I was growing up, I never had a friend for longer than a year. My dad was in the military, so we were often on the move. Feeling the isolation of always being the new kid on the block, I consoled myself with food and grew increasingly heavier as we moved from one town to another. My family and friends told me that I would grow out of my baby-fat stage, and so I just continued to overeat.

I tried to shake off the hurt of being so overweight. When I asked a friend if I could ride her new bike, she said, "No, Kathryn, you would break it down." Another friend would not allow me in her tree house because I could cause it to come crashing down!

I have a great relationship with my mother and father now, and I did back then. They are my best friends, but in looking back, I think the isolation I felt in moving once a year and being in a new town and school fueled my compulsion to overeat.

When I started high school in Maryland, I was doing well in all my classes, but I was known as the jolly overweight girl who played the French horn. I eventually ditched the French horn but not the weight. Starting my first year in college, I weighed 205 pounds.

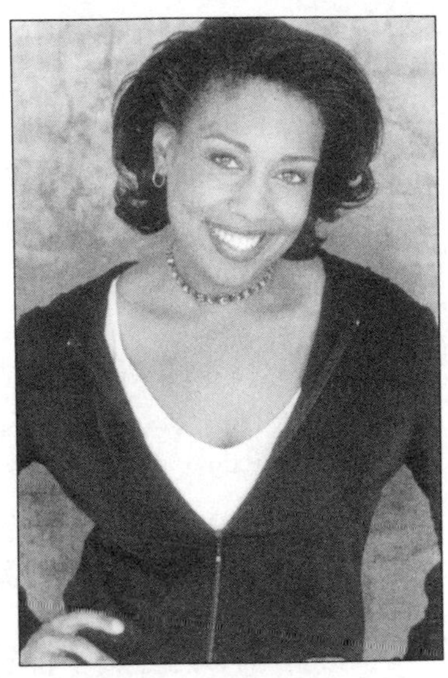

At the end of my freshman year, I was driving three other girls back to school. I had just said, "Something is not right with this car!" when I realized whatever I was doing to steer the car was not working. Just as we approached a bridge, the back of the car spun around. No matter what I did, I could not control the skid. The car seemed to be floating on air and then bounced off the side of the bridge.

I began talking to God, saying, "God, I've lost control, and if You want me to get out of this alive, You are going to have to help me!" I took my hands off the wheel and my feet off the pedals. Within seconds it was over. The car had spun the entire length of the ice-covered bridge and stopped. None of my friends or I was hurt. In fact, I felt that I had been given a second chance in life, but at that time I did not know what to do with it.

My weight was at a relatively stable stage when I started taking acting classes at a new school in Atlanta. After graduating, I moved on to New York, and my career in acting started to take off. Neither my agent or anyone else encouraged me to lose weight. I was able to get work in television commercials because I resembled a popular talk-show host who also had a weight issue. Not realizing that by being overweight I was putting my health in jeopardy, I decided that I needed to stay heavy in order to work.

I received a rude awakening when I tried out for the big time in Los Angeles. When agents there commented on how heavy I was, I went back to New York. Around that time, I noticed that a few stray hairs were growing on my face, but the hair on my head seemed to be thinning. I had gained even more weight and began to have backaches.

When I went back again to give Los Angeles another try, my health problems became even more evident. I was concerned enough to make an appointment with a doctor and was diagnosed with Polycystic Ovarian Syndrome (PCOS). I did a lot of soul searching, because there was not a lot of information available on PCOS at that time. One thing I did know: I had been doing things that were not healthy for anyone, much less for someone with PCOS.

I was ready to do something with that second chance in life that God had given me years before. Although I could not afford to do it, I took a year off from work and concentrated on getting my health back. I remembered a passage about faith from the Bible: "For this slight momentary affliction is preparing us for an eternal weight of glory beyond all measure, because we look not at what can be seen but at what cannot be seen; for what can be seen is temporary, but what cannot be seen is eternal." (2 Cor. 4:17–18) I knew that I needed to focus on my own spirituality and look to God for help.

I prayed, "God, please, please, please help me lose weight!" All of a sudden I had an understanding that God was telling me: "Okay, here is the deal: If you eat right and exercise on a regular basis, I guarantee you that I will take the weight off."

I questioned, "What kind of deal is this?" I wanted God to just make the weight loss happen, but I knew I could not have any better guarantee than a guarantee from God.

Understanding contracts from my work in acting, I decided I would hold up my end of the contract, because I had faith that God would hold up the other end. I ate vegetables that I had not eaten in years, because I was upholding my part of my contract with God. I ate lean cuts of meat and drank glass after glass of water every day. I worked out in the gym at 5:30 in the morning and again at 5:30 that evening. I eliminated sugar and refined carbohydrates from my diet.

Surfing the Internet, I found so much helpful information, learning about the importance of vitamins and phytonutrients and phytochemicals. I read the labels on everything I ate—before I ate! In 14 months, I had lost 90 pounds.

The agents, advertisers, and casting agents in New York were not happy about my weight loss. They would no longer hire me for television commercials. I thought: "God, You have not brought me this far to hang me out to dry. Maybe I'm supposed to go back to Los Angeles and give it one more try."

I packed my suitcase and told my roommate that I would probably be back in a month. In Los Angeles, I immediately started getting calls from people who had heard that I had lost weight. I auditioned for the host of a fitness show, and although I did not get the position of host, I was hired as a correspondent for the show. I covered snowboarding, dogsledding, and cardio-swing classes. Next I was offered 26 episodes on the television show *Vacation Living*.

One month after I got that offer, I received a call from a producer of *Dream Maker*, a television show hosted by Richard Simmons. Because of his dedication to helping people lose weight, Richard was one of my heroes.

I was not as excited about getting the job as I was about having a chance to meet Richard Simmons. When I met with the producers, they seemed mildly unimpressed with me. I told them how much I wanted to meet Richard, and at home that evening, I got a call: I was to meet Richard the next day.

When I arrived at Richard's office for the meeting, there was one more actor being interviewed. I heard

Richard's voice from the next room, a voice that had inspired so many people. As soon as I entered his office, I ran to him and gave him a big hug. We chatted for a while, and then he said, "You're hired."

My job was to deliver dreams to people: One woman who was going blind had always wanted to visit the Grand Canyon. I took her there before she lost her vision. Another dream fulfilled was for a little girl who was so allergic to light that she could not stand even being in the light of an ordinary lightbulb. Her family could not afford a suit made by NASA that would allow her to go outside. Richard and Ed McMahon purchased this suit, and I delivered it.

I have a brand new life since I lost weight. My life has improved and my health has improved also. Women with PCOS have seven times the risk of heart disease, endometriosis, and diabetes. Although the doctors say there is no cure for PCOS, I do not have to be on medication any longer. My symptoms start to creep back when I let myself get stressed out and by eating junk food. But because I remember my contract with God, I get back on track. I eat right and I exercise.

I have shortened my name from Kathryn to Kat, because cats have nine lives. I don't know that I will have nine lives, but I do know that God has given me a second chance at life. I am doing all I know to do to show my appreciation to God.

Today's Message

Energized

I am energized by the presence and power of God within me.

Food, water, and air energize me physically, and I have learned that there is an energy beyond the physical that I can tap into every day through prayer. Prayer energizes me spiritually.

I need a fresh supply of food and water in order to be sustained physically, but because I include prayer and meditation in my daily regimen, I am completely and wholly energized. Physical energy enables me to exist—yet because I am spiritually and physically energized, I thrive. I am whole and holy.

Whenever I do feel a lack of energy, even though I have had food recently, I consider that I might need to nourish myself with prayer. I can connect with a fresh supply of energy every day, several times a day. The life of God within every cell of my body responds to my prayers with a resurgence of energy.

Through the life of God within me, I have a constant source of energy and strength.

"I can do all things through him who strengthens me."
—Philippians 4:13

TODAY'S MESSAGE

Accessories

Thank You, God, for the beauty that adorns my world.

Losing weight has given me the opportunity to replace my wardrobe with new clothes. What an exciting and enjoyable activity this has been! Along with my new clothes, I have bought accessories that add color and uniqueness to my wardrobe.

When I look around me, I see the beauty of the world—the accessories that God has lovingly and generously provided for me and everyone. I see the stars at night that glitter like gemstones. I see lush, green grass in valleys below majestic mountains. Flowing streams sparkle in the sunlight and refresh the world around them. What more could I want than to be at one with these natural and divine adornments of the world?

When I think about the physical changes I have gone through, I know without a doubt that I have also changed spiritually. I know that my life has been enriched by my new awareness of the beauty and goodness of God.

"But the Lord made the heavens. Honor and majesty are before him; strength and beauty are in his sanctuary."
—Psalms 96:6

Today's Message

Rewards of Today

—◆—

I reap the rewards of God's gifts of newfound confidence and courage, peace and poise.

The rewards of today come in many shapes and sizes and in ways that are completely intangible. I may see enticements to be or do more. Some advertisers may tell me that I need to use a certain product in order to be a better person mentally, physically, or emotionally. But when I look within my heart, I know the rewards of my personal relationship with God.

I can pray and turn to God for guidance in knowing what to do for inspiration to make changes and for strength to do anything I need to do. As I look to God for help in every situation, I reap the rewards of God's love in all that I do. God's love teaches me to love myself, to see myself as God sees me—wise and loving, confident and whole.

I find the rewards of today in letting go of the regrets of the past. Anything I have done in the past no longer has any hold on me. I am living in this present moment and reaping the rewards of living for today.

"Your Father who sees in secret will reward you."
—Matthew 6:2

Today's Message

Standing Firm

I stand firm in my faith in God's love for me and attention to me.

Others may not always agree with the decisions I make, but I pray that I always act on God's guidance, for it is meant solely for me. I stand firm in the faith that God knows what is best for me.

Although I cannot see into the future, I know that the choices I make today may affect my health and well-being in the next few days or even years from now. So I rely on the wisdom of God to be the source for my decisions.

There is no situation or place that I can ever be that could possibly be beyond the power of my Creator's love for me and attention to me. So I stand firm in my faith in God to direct me. With every decision I make, I am following a divine plan.

Within all situations, through all times, I have a deep desire to live my life fully aware that God is working with me and through me, guiding me on my way.

"Surely then you will lift up your face . . . you will be secure, and will not fear."
—Job 11:15

TODAY'S MESSAGE

Revelation

God is continually revealing the happy, whole, and loving person that I am.

Being consistent with my routines day after day, I may find that I am so absorbed in the act of doing that I may not recognize the results that I am achieving. Since my regimen of diet and exercise has been going on for a while, I may not have noticed subtle differences in the way my clothes fit or how much easier I breathe during a brisk walk.

Today I expand my awareness and become an observer of myself and of what has taken place over the last few months. This total view offers me a revelation about myself: I have changed, and my changes have been for the better. I feel whole and at peace, because I am now living from the joy within my soul. I realize that one of my greatest purposes for being is to share the joy and love within me with others.

I have experienced a divine revelation about myself—I am happy, whole, and filled with the love of God.

**"Into your hand I commit my spirit;
you have redeemed me, O Lord, faithful God."
—Psalms 31:5**

Today's Message

Blessing Food

I bless my food and my food blesses me.

I want to choose and prepare food that will bless me. One way I am reminded to choose and prepare the best is to bless my food. My silent blessing as I choose food in a grocery store or the blessing I speak aloud before a meal does not reduce the calories or fat content of food, but because I am so aware of my selections and the way I cook, I am sending a message to myself: What I choose and the way I prepare it helps me stay slim.

I do not eat just anything because I am in a rush and hungry. I eat what nourishes me without loading up with excess calories that would only be stored as fat in my body. I am thinking and praying my way through the day, and because I do, I make wise, nutritional selections of food choices and recipes.

My very thoughts about my health are prayers that prepare me to stay healthy and energetic. No extra calories mean no extra pounds.

"They had also a few small fish; and after blessing them, he ordered that these too should be distributed. They ate and were filled."

—Mark 8:7–8

MEDITATION

Nourishing My Soul

Each day, I faithfully nourish my soul through prayer and meditation.

I gently ease into a sacred time of prayer, closing my eyes and turning within. Here I nourish my soul through an intimate time with God. As my thoughts are stilled, the gentle, loving voice of God resonates throughout my being:

"Dear one, I have created so much beauty and diversity in the world—one creation at a time. You are one of My unique creations, and yet you share a common bond with all life. My spirit within all is that bond."

As God's words move into my subconscious, I no longer feel an attachment to any outside influence. I am soaring with the freedom of Spirit. When I return to the present, I bring that sense of spiritual nourishment with me.

I remember to dedicate time each day to nourishing my soul through prayer and meditation.

"Beloved, I pray that all may go well with you and that you may be in good health, just as it is well with your soul."
—3 John 1:2

◆ *Journal* ◆

Date: ____

My weight: ____________________________________

If I am having a difficult day,
I do not seek solice in food.

Instead I ______________________________________

Today's Message

Planning

—◆—

I am planning to stay trim and energized by relying on the wisdom and inspiration of my Creator.

Life would seem so much easier if I didn't have to do so much planning. The reality, however, is that thinking about and arranging a goal or an event can be rewarding. Whether I am planning a party, a vacation, or a meal, planning can be as enjoyable as I allow it to be. Creating a guest list, choosing a travel route, or picking the freshest ingredients for a new recipe all involve me and how I can help bring about the results I desire.

So I accept that even though my scales no longer cause the red flag marked "diet" to pop up, I still plan my meals and snacks so that I get the optimum nutritional benefits but keep my calorie intake at a reasonable level. I am into planning and glad that I am, because this is the way I ensure that I stay trim and energized. I continue to plan for a healthy body and lifestyle by relying on the wisdom and inspiration of my Creator.

"With all wisdom and insight he has made known to us the mystery of his will, according to his good pleasure that he set forth in Christ, as a plan for the fullness of time."
—Ephesians 1:8–10

Today's Message

Still Evolving

Each day I am evolving into someone greater than I was the day before.

I am a work in progress, and God, the Master Artist, is continually adding depth, definition, and highlights to the canvas of my life. Only the Master knows what the finished piece will be like, but one thing I know is that I am a masterpiece created by the divine Creator.

Each day is a new adventure for me. I may not know what the day holds when I arise each morning, but with my newfound energy and vigor, I am prepared to enjoy life by living each day with the fullness of Spirit.

With each passing day, I am evolving. If challenges should arise, God will see me through them. I think of myself as being refined by spiritual understanding. Awake to Spirit each day, I am continually evolving into someone greater than I was even the day before.

"For you, O Lord, are my hope,
my trust, O Lord, from my youth."
—Psalms 71:5

Today's Message

Breaking the Cycle

—◆—

With faith in God, I leave old habits behind and stand on the mountaintop of success.

When I am feeling good about my weight loss and am able to maintain a weight I am comfortable with, I feel as though I am standing on a mountaintop. Because I want to continue to maintain my weight, I take responsibility for my success by breaking the cycle of losing and then gaining weight.

If remaining within my weight range seems to be a battle, I once again rely on ways in which I have been especially successful at losing weight, and I trust in God for the strength to continue. I may remind myself of tips about food or exercise that worked before. If the same techniques are not effective the second or third time, I look for new, more successful ways.

I know that God will help me break the cycle of poor eating habits, negative thinking, or any behavior that is not beneficial. As I spend time in prayer, I am lifted out of the valley of old habits and onto the mountaintop of success.

"God, the Lord, is my strength; he makes my feet like the feet of a deer, and makes me tread upon the heights."
—Habakkuk 3:19

Today's Message

Easy Day

This is an easy day, for spiritual understanding is helping me understand myself and my actions.

One of the most important things I have learned is that sometimes I make things harder for myself—in the way I *think* myself into doing or not doing something. For instance: Why would I choose to make my day harder when there is an easier way of accomplishing something? The answer is that I don't. I am not always looking for the easy way out, but occasionally I need to give myself a break. And I do!

Through spiritual understanding, I gain a better perspective of myself and my actions—what benefits others and me. My willpower may be tested when I eat out, but the truth is my willpower is tested every day. So I stock up on low-calorie flavorful foods and keep high-calorie foods out of the house.

I help create my day, and make it shine with accomplishment, knowing that the next day is another opportunity to be easy on myself.

"A scoffer seeks wisdom in vain, but knowledge is easy for one who understands."
—Proverbs 14:6

Today's Message

Power of Prayer

Prayer serves as a bridge, linking me—heart and soul—with the presence of God.

Even though I am fully aware that divine order is actively at work in my life and in the universe, I still pray. Prayer is a powerful way that I feel a oneness with God, for prayer is a bridge that links my awareness to God's presence.

As I pray, I become more enlightened, so that I am fully aware: ". . . for God all things are possible." (Mk. 10:27) I feel a surge of joy as I imagine all of the unlimited possibilities that lie before me.

Because I would never want to limit those divine possibilities with my own thinking, I do not pray for a particular outcome. Instead, I pray with gratitude, affirming that God is answering my every need and desire in the right time and in the right way.

In prayer, I receive confirmation that I am linking my heart and soul with the mighty presence of God.

**"I saw the Lord always before me,
for he is at my right hand so that I
will not be shaken."
—Acts 2:25**

Today's Message

Thinking It Over

As I reflect on God's wisdom, I receive insight about being the healthy, happy person I am meant to be.

Sometimes when I think my progress is going smoothly, I may be tripped up by a little surprise. Before I take a step that may not be consistent with my commitment to take good care of myself, I stop and think it over. I take a God break and breathe deeply. This is my signal to myself that I need to consult God for the guidance that will enable me to do the right thing.

Such reflective pauses give me an opportunity to tap into the source of wisdom and understanding that I need at times like this. During a few brief moments, I can turn my attention to the presence of God within me. God is a loving presence that provides a fount of insight and understanding, showing me what I need to know to rise above any temptation or setback.

Placing my full attention on God bolsters my faith and determination. With God to guide and uphold me, I can be the healthy, happy person I am meant to be.

"Think over what I say, for the Lord will give you understanding in all things."
—2 Timothy 2:7

MEDITATION

Temple of God

I am a temple of God.

Because prayer and meditation are an integral part of my life, I set aside a room in my home where I can concentrate solely on entering into a time of silence. This place is quiet—a place where I can play soothing music in the background to center my mind. A favorite aroma helps me go within to that center of peace at the core of my being.

I easily forget the outside world as I settle in, closing my eyes and opening my thoughts to God. I take several deep cleansing breaths and repeat to myself: *My body is a temple of God*.

As I reach that inner place of absolute peace, I feel a oneness with God's presence. *My mind is a temple of God*. Because I am born of Spirit, I am attuned to the guiding, loving presence of God. *My soul is a temple of God*. It is in going within that I am fully aware of God and that I am a temple of God.

"So acknowledge today and take to heart that the Lord is God in heaven above and on earth beneath; there is no other."
—Deuteronomy 4:39

◆ *Journal* ◆

Date: ________________________________

My weight: ____________________________

I have left my old, negative habits behind and have developed new, positive ones that benefit me.

My new habits include ____________________

____

____

____

____

____

____

____

____

____

____

Today's Message

Checking In

The love of God encourages me to be strong and successful.

From time to time, I "check in" at the scales to be sure I am maintaining my desired weight. Weighing regularly helps me know whether I need to adjust the way I am eating and what I am eating.

If I am concerned about gaining weight, I may keep a journal that provides me with an overview of my daily routines and when I was especially successful at maintaining or losing weight.

I may make a checklist of my success by asking myself what I have done that worked best and what I have learned about my eating and exercise habits. I certainly want to make good use of the positive new habits I have acquired. I take time to reflect on my success and give thanks for God's ever-present love.

I do what I can, such as checking my weight, reading my journal, and examining my checklist; however, I know that I can trust God's steadfast love to uphold me every day and encourage me throughout all my days.

"I trust in the steadfast love of God forever and ever." —Psalms 52:8

Today's Message

What I Treasure

What I treasure most is God's presence, a holy presence that satisfies me.

The material, tangible objects I collect are only things, not what I truly treasure in life. Today, tomorrow, or the next day, something may happen, and I no longer have them. They may have been lost, sold, or broken.

There is a Presence that I do treasure above all else—a holy Presence that is always with me through all situations and at all times. This priceless treasure is God, and the glory of God's creativity shines in me and everywhere in creation as life and intelligence.

I do not need a miracle to occur in my life to prove the existence of God. Each day subtle clues serve as reminders that God is everywhere present.

When I see the sparkling canopy of a midnight sky, I do not question whether the universe was divinely created. I question how any person could look at such magnitude and beauty and not believe. I feel a sense of gratitude and wonder when I consider the treasure that God is and how God satisfies my every need.

"God will fully satisfy every need of yours according to his riches."
—Philippians 4:19

Today's Message
My Model

—◆—

I give thanks for all the people who have influenced me and blessed me.

There are so many important people in my life, people who have influenced me personally, professionally, and spiritually. Thinking of these people has inspired me in my achievements and been my impetus whenever I may have felt the desire to give up.

Role models are important, for they remind me of what can be achieved. As I continue to maintain my weight and health, I remember that I am a role model for others. Sharing my successes and even my failures may be helpful to others. By sharing, I am a channel of inspiration and blessings to those who are working toward goals.

I give thanks for the many role models in my life and for the ways in which they have influenced me. Some are family and friends who have been there for me all the while and some are strangers who will never even know the impact they have left upon me. Each of them has helped me overcome obstacles and be successful.

"Show yourself in all respects a model of good works."
—Titus 2:7

TODAY'S MESSAGE

Readjustments

I am making readjustments so that I continue to follow a divine plan of enhancing myself and my life.

Has losing weight made a new person of me? My expectations of what I would look like and how I would feel may not have been fulfilled.

I'm sure that I have more confidence, but I doubt that my IQ went up as remarkably as my weight went down. I have gained strength and flexibility through my exercise program, but my body may not be the perfect shape that I had envisioned it would be.

Maybe what I need to do is to readjust my thinking so that I realize that life itself is about change. Through diet and exercise, prayer and meditation, I am achieving important changes in myself. I am grateful to God for life, and I am showing my gratitude by being willing to treat myself with the reverence and honor that a creation of God's deserves. Every week or so, I check my expectations and my habits so that I can and do readjust them to fit in with a divine plan.

"Cease straying, my child, from the words of knowledge, in order that you may hear instruction."
—Proverbs 19:27

Today's Message

What Works

—◆—

Day after day, the spirit of God helps me sustain my commitment to living with a positive, healthy outlook.

I have come so far in living a healthier life. Whenever I need to feel stronger about my determination to persevere, I think back to when I was able to meet a challenge successfully. Remembering what helps me succeed keeps me steady on my journey of healthful living.

Moment by moment, the spirit of God within enables me to move through any difficulty. I know that I don't have to struggle to keep my commitment to myself. I release any need to control matters, and I allow the spirit of God to do what it does best. God's spirit guides my thoughts and actions, reinforces my inner resolve, and strengthens my body.

How fortunate I am to have such marvelous help in maintaining my commitment! I am able to sustain not only my physical well-being but also my positive outlook, an outlook that sees God's spirit at work in me and all that concerns me.

"Commit your work to the Lord,
and your plans will be established."
—Proverbs 16:3

TODAY'S MESSAGE

Variety

Using a variety of foods and flavors, I eat right and I am also satisfied.

I use my God-given wisdom to think my way out of becoming bored with good food. Something as simple as enhancing the taste of familiar food with spices adds to the variety of my menu. A portion of plain green beans takes on added flavor and texture when I add a few slivered almonds.

Often it is not what I eat but how much I eat that could cause me to gain weight, so I pay attention to portions. Every once in a while I taste a dessert so I don't feel so deprived that I eventually break down and go overboard. Other times I let fresh, juicy fruit be a sweet dessert that comes straight from nature.

There is so much variety in the natural foods that God has created, and there is so much creativity open to me in being satisfied while eating right.

"I know that there is nothing better for them than to be happy and enjoy themselves as long as they live; moreover, it is God's gift that all should eat and drink and take pleasure in all their toil."
—Ecclesiastes 3:12–13

MEDITATION

Serendipity

Today is a day of serendipity: a day in which I will find something of great value.

For a few moments I retreat from the world around me. This is a time for me to be still and silent. I open my mind and heart to revelations from God. There is nothing for me to do or say; I just receive.

Scenes of discovery appear in my mind's eye as I rest. I recognize times of serendipity: times when I found something of great value when I was not consciously seeking it. When I prepared healthy low-fat meals because *I* wanted to lose weight, I also helped my family reduce their fat intake. When I felt good about my accomplishments, I shared those good feelings in my relationships, which actually improved my communication with and enjoyment of others.

Slowly I return my thoughts to my surroundings and give thanks that many more moments of serendipity await my discovery.

"Happy are the people to whom such blessings fall; happy are the people whose God is the Lord."
—Psalms 144:15

◆ *Journal* ◆

Date: ________________________________

My weight: ____________________________

My positive attitude inspires me
to remember to thank God
for my blessings.

I am thankful for people, fresh air, and ______

____

____

____

____

____

____

____

____

____

____

TODAY'S MESSAGE

Celebrating Holidays

Holidays offer me great opportunities to show how creative I can be.

Special occasions may test my resolve to stay with my healthy eating plan. Holidays seem to revolve around preparing and eating food. Relatives and friends labor over their special recipes and may be offended if others do not eat a second helping.

I can be both honest and creative in passing on seconds by saying, "That was so good, I just want to sit back and savor the wonderful flavor for a while." Or, "I am so satisfied and comfortably full right now that I don't want to ruin the experience by overindulging."

I can also be creative in adding to holiday times with family and friends. Sharing favorite stories with each other or looking at picture albums of us in the "good old days" revives warm memories and adds a special joy to these gatherings. I am creative in bringing a special, loving touch to our times together.

"This day shall be a day of remembrance for you. You shall celebrate it as a festival to the Lord; throughout your generations you shall observe it as a perpetual ordinance."
—Exodus 12:14

Today's Message

Lately

—◆—

I have made so much progress that a new me has emerged.

As I think about all that has occurred over the last few months and the change in the way I look, I wonder: How has my attitude changed lately? Do I have greater expectations about myself and my life? What habits and thoughts have I released or held on to?

As I look back, I can see the progress I have made—physically, spiritually, and mentally. I understand that lately I am a happier person and a more spiritual person. I am a person who is not only satisfied with life; I also find great joy in life.

A new me has emerged, a new me that not only feels lighter physically but spiritually as well. I feel as if a burden has been lifted from me, a burden of negative thoughts and habits. What a realization this is! How great it is to know how much I have grown in understanding of myself and to experience true freedom.

Like a butterfly that has emerged from its cocoon, a new me has emerged from old thoughts and patterns.

"See, I am making all things new."
—Revelation 21:5

Today's Message

Keeping the Faith

—◆—

I have faith in God and faith in what God can do through me.

Starting off by having faith that I can accomplish something may not be so much of a challenge for me, but keeping my faith over a period of time may be.

I knew I could lose weight, and I have invested my time and effort in doing just that. Now it is time for me to keep that faith ongoing so that I keep the weight off.

There will always be ups and downs in life, but my weight is something I can keep stable. I am the one who puts food into my mouth, exercises, and decides what my day will be.

Having faith in God is never a problem for me, but I also need to have faith in myself. I do when I recognize that I am God's creation and as such, I am fully capable of handling the simple and complex nature of life.

I am keeping my faith in God and keeping my faith in what God can do through me.

"Then Jesus answered her, 'Woman, great is your faith! Let it be done for you as you wish.' And her daughter was healed instantly."
—Matthew 15:28

Today's Message

Getting Acquainted

In a spirit of friendship and fellowship, I share with and learn from others.

I have heard that there is strength in numbers, and I believe that when I surround myself with people of like minds, I strengthen my own resolve to stay with a program.

Although there is a special love between my family and me, and my longtime friends and me, I have made new acquaintances within a group who have helped me. I hope I have helped them also.

Getting acquainted with others and talking about weight and lifestyle practices may not have been all that easy, but it has certainly been worthwhile. In a spirit of friendship and fellowship, we have shared the common purpose of attaining greater health and maintaining that health.

These are important acquaintances, and I want to check in with them in the future, continuing to share with them and learn from them.

"Some friends play at friendship but a true friend sticks closer than one's nearest kin."
—Proverbs 18:24

Today's Message

What a Relief!

—◆—

What a sense of relief I feel knowing that the steps I am taking toward improving my health are working!

I have been making healthy choices for some time now, and these choices come naturally to me. When I prepare a meal or choose items from a menu, what a relief it is to know that I am in control.

Because of the past choices I have made, I not only look good, I feel good as well. Now that I know how good it feels to live a healthy lifestyle, I want to hold on to that feeling, keeping it in mind whether I am eating alone or with others.

When I shop at a grocery store, what a sense of relief I feel as I focus on those foods that are good for me. Junk food no longer appeals to me, and I can and do steer clear of it.

Trying on a smaller-size outfit and discovering that it fits perfectly is a relief and a joy. Because I look good in it and feel comfortable wearing it, I may not hesitate buying it—even though it's not on sale.

What a relief I feel in knowing that the steps I am taking toward improving my health are working!

"To set the mind on the Spirit is life and peace."
—Romans 8:6

Today's Message

Graduation Day

—◆—

I am filled with confidence, for I have graduated from learning how to control my weight to controlling it.

Graduating from a high school or college may have boosted my confidence and given me a sense of purpose and accomplishment.

I am celebrating a different kind of graduation of late: I have graduated from learning how I can control my weight to actually doing it. I am putting some well-earned knowledge to practice every day.

I may not have a diploma to display, but my trimmer shape, my increased energy, and my greater confidence are confirmation that I learned and have put that learning to good use. The light of wisdom shines from my eyes, and I begin each day with a sense of accomplishment.

I am confident that I can and will continue to make right choices and do whatever I need to do to maintain and even improve my health and well-being.

"The light shines in the darkness,
and the darkness did not overcome it."
—John 1:5

Meditation

The Rest of My Life

Immersed in the presence of God, I see the road before me and realize that I am prepared for life.

Gently, quietly I release all awareness of what is going on around me. I let my body slowly settle into a comfortable position, and then I close my eyes. In a time of inner contemplation, I immerse myself in the presence of God.

I am at peace and focused on this sacred moment. I feel, more than hear, my Creator assuring me that I am loved unconditionally. I understand that on my life journey, God is always my companion and the source of all the good I could ever need or want—and even more.

As though through a mist, I see the road before me and realize that I am prepared to live life with understanding and in health. The wisdom that created the universe protects me, guides me, and inspires me—now and all the rest of my life.

"Surely goodness and mercy shall follow me
all the days of my life,
and I shall dwell in the house of the Lord
my whole life long."
—Psalms 23:6

◆ *Journal* ◆

Date: ______________________________

My weight: ______________________________

Maintaining my ideal weight is a lifetime commitment. To keep this commitment, I continue with healthy eating patterns and exercise on a regular basis.

I am also committed to ____________________

____

____

____

____

____

____

____

____

____

Just 30 minutes of aerobic exercise 4 days a week promotes loss of body fat and decreases blood pressure, blood sugar, anxiety, depression, and insomnia.

◆

SOURCE: Susan Smith Jones, Health Unlimited

One Step at a Time

By Candi Foster

In 1984, after a lifetime of being overweight, I decided to take control of my life and change at least that one aspect. Making the decision to lose weight was the easy part. What followed required more effort and lots of determination.

In July of that year, I walked into my first Weight Watchers meeting not expecting to join—only wanting to see if it was something I thought would help me. The attending clerk convinced me that I might as well stay since I was already there. I knew the program did work for others, because my mother had shed more than 60 pounds by following the program. Would it work for me? Only if I was willing to try. Over the next year or so, I lost enough to wear a size 16—something I had not been able to do since I was a teenager.

Then events of my life got in my way. I went through a divorce, changed jobs three times, and helped my best friend pack and move clear across the country. In one year, I attended the funerals of three of my grandparents. There were just too many other things on my mind to have to deal with thinking about food, too. I went back to eating my version of the four basic food groups: fried food, fast food, breads, and desserts.

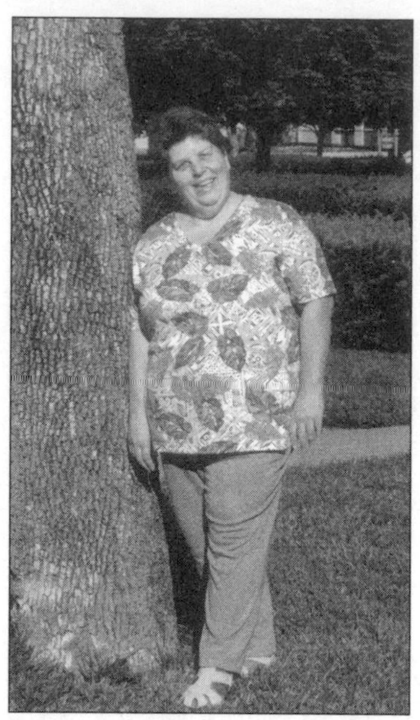

Off and on, I tried on my own to lose weight. I even went back to Weight Watchers a few times but would get discouraged and quit. Each time I joined and quit, I put on more weight than I had taken off.

Gaining pound after pound of weight, I reached the point that breathing itself was an effort. I could not sleep at night. I could not stand up long enough to fry an egg and had to order clothes from a catalog in order to find any large enough for me. Walking was nearly impossible. In fact, any kind of movement was a special kind of torture. I was depressed, angry, and could almost feel my waist expanding daily. Words like *exercise, self-esteem,* and *control* were not a part of my vocabulary. I truly felt that I was caught in an undertow of despair that was pulling me deeper and deeper into a place I was not likely to survive.

When my job was terminated and I had no recourse but to move in with my parents and start over, my anger and self-pity blossomed right along with my weight. In the middle of it all, though, God was working through me and my life to establish new beginnings and reveal many wonderful blessings. In a short time, I was led to a place of employment where I do work that I truly love, and I work with people who are kind, loving, supportive, and believe in the power of prayer.

As I spent more time in this positive environment, I began to notice a shift in my own thinking and self-awareness. My prayers changed from pleading and expecting overnight miracles to: "God, just show me what to do and help me do it."

One of my favorite Bible verses has always been "I can do all things through Christ who strengthens me." I began to repeat that verse to myself over and over throughout the day. Any time feelings of defeat and discouragement came up, I repeated my simple prayer. Little by little, I noticed my attitude toward myself and others changing.

Seeds of inspiration took root in my mind and sprouted into visions of manageable, easy-to-do changes in actions and attitude. I began thinking, "I CAN do this and I WILL do this."

When a friend mentioned going to Weight Watchers, it was as though I heard God whisper to me, "This is it, and you are ready. We can do this." So I joined Weight Watchers again. This time it was with the conviction that God would help me each step of the way.

It had taken me 16 years to get to this point, but I was

ready now to make the necessary commitment, even though by this time taking off the extra pounds would not be a short-term project.

With the encouragement of others in the weekly meetings I attended, and a 4-pound weight loss the first week, I knew that I was now well on my way to making positive changes in my lifestyle.

Eventually, I reached a plateau where I was losing little or nothing each week even though I continued to eat properly. Exercise was the one aspect of weight loss that I had always ignored. I really expected to be able to reach my goal weight without exercising, and told myself I would exercise when I was thin enough to do it easily. But, I had asked God to show me what to do, and little by little, I found myself doing things I had not done before. I began to walk up the stairs—one flight only at first—instead of taking the elevator. I parked farther away from the door at work or at the mall so I would have to walk a longer distance.

A little at a time, I found ways to increase my activity. Knowing that if I was going to exercise I would have to do it early in the day, I set aside a special time every morning to ride a stationary bike. At first, I could only manage about 15 minutes at a time. Slowly, I increased the amount of time to a half hour. Then I added 10-minute walking breaks twice a day and joined a women-only exercise/fitness facility. I soon realized that I was spending almost an hour a day exercising! And each step of the way, a still, small voice within urged me on and encouraged me to keep up the good work.

At the end of one month, I had lost a total of 13 inches and 8 pounds. My enthusiasm soared as I mentally recorded one more success.

The exercise and walking produce other benefits as well. Those quiet times alone are free from distraction and an ideal time to communicate with God. After a morning walk, I am peaceful, energized, and ready to greet the day with a strong positive outlook. After a 30-minute workout, I feel better about myself and ready to make one more day a successful day.

Daily, I grew stronger both physically and emotionally. I watched the scales register a steady decline in my weight. Ten pounds. Twenty-five. Fifty. Seventy-five pounds in the first year. In 18 months, I lost 100 pounds. With each drop in the scale, my degree of self-confidence rose another notch. My energy level increased, and my outlook on life improved 100 percent! At last, healthy eating habits and regular exercise had become routine.

One step at a time, one little change at a time, one goal at a time, I stepped from the edge of despondency to the pinnacle of success.

I cannot take total credit for my weight-loss success. My family, friends, and coworkers are an important part of the formula. The compliments of those who have seen me at my heaviest and who daily witness my progress encourage me to keep going and provide me with incentives to reach my goal. I am setting an example for others by staying committed and working steadily toward that goal.

I have not yet reached my goal weight. I still have a long way to go. I know that I will always have to make a conscious effort to lose or maintain my weight, and that it may not always be easy. Occasionally, challenges and unexpected events may tempt me to stray from the path that leads to success. That is why it is important for me to establish new, stronger habits of healthy eating, to exercise daily, and to keep a positive mental attitude. I want to face each day of the rest of my life with the understanding that I can succeed. I am determined to reach a weight that is right for me and to maintain that weight.

If there are times that I do not lose as much as I had hoped, I remind myself of how much I have already accomplished and ask myself what I can learn from this experience. It is disappointing to gain when I have tried so hard to lose, but I realize that there are many factors—some beyond my control—that contribute to the numbers that appear when I step on the scale.

And if I am tempted to feel sorry for myself because I am not losing as fast as I would like, I think of how good it feels to be able to walk without pain, to shop for clothes in a department store, and do other things I have not been able to do for a long time. I picture myself as I want to be and know that I will achieve that vision. I trust God to guide me, for as my constant companion, God will be with me every step of the way.

I am walking toward new horizons of possibility!

About the Featured Authors

Kat Carney shed 90 pounds in 14 months through proper diet, nutritional education, and lots of exercise. To keep herself motivated, she tore weight-loss success stories out of fitness magazines and hung them on a wall so that she was surrounded by "success." She shared her own success story when she was hired as a correspondent on cable's "Fit: Resort and Spa." That same year, she worked next to weight-loss guru Richard Simmons on the nationally syndicated television show *Dream Maker*. In January 2000, Kat decided to put all the stories she had collected in one place: www.TheWeighWeWere.com. She sends out free "Daily InspirWeighTional" quotes via e-mail to thousands of people. Kat was asked to tell her story on the Discovery Channel's new "Health" network and 5 months later was hired to host their new prime-time series *The Body Invaders*. In June 2000, after receiving thousands of e-mails from women around the world with Polycystic Ovarian Syndrome, Kat launched www.SoulCysters.com, the largest online community for women diagnosed with PCOS. Kat currently works as a health news anchor for CNN Headline News.

Candi Foster taught English and journalism at a high school in southwestern Missouri for 10 years, worked as a copywriter for a national real estate magazine, and served as manager of a college bookstore. Candi has worked at Unity School of Christianity since 1996, and her interests include animals, traveling, crocheting, and reading. A dedicated Weight Watchers member,

Candi lives in a suburb near Unity Village with her dog, Lucy, and her cat, Toby.

Tamara Guilliams continues to work at Unity School of Christianity. She lives in Raytown, Missouri, where she enjoys studying metaphysics, taking long walks, sewing, gardening, watching comedies, and living life with her friends and her teenage sons, Wesley David and Alexander Thomas. In addition, Tamara is preparing workshops on the topics of healing and weight release, based on the principles she practices. She also plans on writing a book so that others may learn from her experiences. Tamara may be contacted at P.O. Box 285, Lee's Summit, MO 64063.

Edie Hand is a business owner, radio personality, actress, author, mother, and the epitome of today's multi-dimensional woman. Edie has been a guest on both the radio and television talk-show circuits. She has appeared on *The Sally Jessy Raphael Show, Live! with Regis and Kathie Lee,* TNN, CNBC, and the Home Shopping Network. She has also appeared on *As the World Turns,* as cohost of *Total Wellness for Women* with Dr. Judy Kuriansky, and as cohost of a television special with legendary songwriter/publisher Buddy Killen. As a cousin of the late Elvis Presley, Edie has coauthored three books on Elvis with cousin Donna Presley Early and is the author of *Recipes for Life: A Cookbook for the Heart and Soul with Edie & Friends.* She is the national spokesperson for Bestfoods Mazola canola oil. For more information, please call (205) 648-8944, or visit www.ediehand.com or www.ediehandfoundation.org.

Peggy Pifer has served in Silent Unity, the prayer ministry of Unity School of Christianity, since 1978. She has been writing for Unity since 1984 and is currently the editor of Silent Unity's Composition Department. Peggy and her husband make their home in Lee's Summit, Missouri.

Susan Smith Jones, Ph.D., has made extraordinary contributions in the fields of optimum health, fitness, and human potential. Selected as 1 of 10 "Healthy American Fitness Leaders" by the President's Council on Physical Fitness and Sports, Susan is the author of 10 books including Pulitzer Prize–nominated *Choose to Live Peacefully, Wired to Meditate: Making the Connection with Your Divine Source*, and *A Fresh Start: Sure-Fire Tips & Recipes to Accelerate Fat Loss & Restore Youthful Vitality*. She holds a Ph.D. in health sciences and has been a fitness instructor to students, staff, and faculty at UCLA for the past 30 years. Susan has written more than 500 magazine articles and appears regularly on radio and television talk shows around the country. She is also founder and president of Health Unlimited, a Los Angeles–based consulting firm dedicated to the advancement of peaceful and balanced living, personal empowerment, and health education. For more information on Susan and her work, log onto www.susansmithjones.com, or to order her books, call (800) 843-5743 Monday thru Friday from 8:00 A.M. to 5:00 P.M. (PST).

ABOUT THE *DAILY WORD* EDITORS

The *Daily Word* editors have also coauthored and coedited *Daily Word: Love, Inspiration, and Guidance for Everyone; Daily Word Prayer Journal; Daily Word for Women; Daily Word for Families; Daily Word for Healing;* and *Daily Word for Couples.*

Colleen Zuck has been editor of *Daily Word* magazine since 1985. She also served as editor of *Wee Wisdom,* the longest continuously published magazine for children in the United States. She lives with her husband, Bill, in rural Missouri.

Elaine Meyer has served in the Silent Unity ministry of Unity School of Christianity since 1987 and is the assistant editor of *Daily Word* magazine. She is also a published poet and writer. She resides with her husband, Dale, and their daughter, Caitlin, in rural Missouri.